MELANOMA DIET COOKBOOK

Optimal Diet To Boost The Immune And Reduce Inflammation Including 170+ Nutrient Recipes To Maintain Healthy Living and Management of Skin Cancer Treatment.

All intellectual property rights are reserved.

Copyright © 2023 [Rebbeca N. Stokes]

Without the publisher's prior written consent, no part of this publication may be copied, distributed or transmitted in any way Including by photocopying, recording or other electronic or mechanical methods with the exception of brief quotations used in critical reviews and other noncommercial uses allowed by copyright law.

TABLE OF CONTENT

CHAPTER 10: WEEKLY MEAL PLAN FOR MELANOMA SURVIVORS........179

CHAPTER 1: INTRODUCTION

A culinary voyage awaits in the sun-kissed realm where flavor meets health, a journey that surpasses the ordinary flowing across the pages of a Melanoma Diet Cookbook. Consider a tapestry of bright foods each chosen not only for their culinary prowess but also for their ability to embrace wellbeing. As the sun sets join us on a gourmet excursion designed for individuals looking for more than simply a meal but a means to fuel and fortify against the shadows of melanoma. This cookbook is more than just a compilation of recipes it is a monument to the harmonious union of taste and tenacity. Let us embark on a culinary journey that will celebrate life one tasty chapter at a time.

OVERVIEW OF MELANOMA

Melanoma, the most dangerous of skin malignancies develops from the uncontrolled proliferation of pigment-producing cells known as melanocytes. Melanoma unlike its cousins has the ability to penetrate surrounding tissues and spread to distant organs making early identification and understanding critical.

This aggressive cancer generally appears as an irregular mole or lesion that changes shape, size or color. UV radiation exposure, hereditary factors and a history of severe sunburns all contribute to its formation.

Melanoma's gravity stems not only from its skin-deep impact but also from its ability to spread entering lymph nodes and organs and posing a severe threat to one's health. Vigilance, education and timely intervention become critical in navigating the complex melanoma terrain.

IMPORTANCE OF NUTRITION IN MELANOMA CARE

Nutrition emerges as a powerful ally in the fight against melanoma influencing not only overall well-being but also playing a crucial part in the holistic care of patients dealing with this formidable foe.

1. Nutrition functions as a frontline defense at the cellular level. Antioxidant-rich foods such as fruits and vegetables provide the body with the resources it needs to neutralize free radicals thus lowering the chance of cellular damage which can lead to the development of melanoma.

2. Immune Support: A well-balanced diet can help boost the immune system, the body's natural defense against cancer. Nutrient-dense diets, vitamins and minerals boost immune responses assisting in the detection and elimination of aberrant cells such as melanoma.

3. Inflammation Control: Chronic inflammation is a well-known contributor to cancer progression. Optimal nutrition which includes anti-inflammatory ingredients such as omega-3 fatty acids and some spices may help to manage inflammation and create an environment that is less conducive to melanoma growth.

4. Skin Health: Nutrition has a direct impact on skin health, and a diet high in particular nutrients can help maintain skin integrity. This includes meals high in vitamins C and E which are necessary for skin regeneration and protection against UV-induced damage which is a significant risk factor for melanoma.

5. Mitigation of Side Effects: During melanoma treatment, patients may experience side effects that affect their nutritional intake. Diets must be tailored to specific concerns such as loss of appetite or digestive issues in order to retain strength and vitality during the healing process.

TYPES OF MELANOMA

1. Melanoma with Superficial Spreading:

The most common form, distinguished by its proclivity to spread across the skin's surface before infiltrating deeper layers.

Appearance: Irregular borders, a variety of colors and an asymmetrical shape are all frequent characteristics.

2. Melanoma with Nodules:

Characteristics: Rapid vertical development, entering the skin faster than other varieties.

Appearance: Usually appears as a raised mass of a uniform color usually black or dark brown.

3. Melanoma Lentigo Maligna:

Characteristics: Slowly develops over time, particularly in sun-exposed places. Prolonged sun exposure has been linked to this condition.

Displays as a wide flat area with irregular boundaries and a variety of colors.

4. Melanoma of the Acral Lentiginous Type:

Characteristics: Usually found on the palms, soles or behind the nails in people with darker skin tones.

Appearance: Usually appears as a black patch or streak that is unrelated to UV exposure.

5. Melanoma of the Amelanotic Skin:

Characteristics: It is unusual in that it lacks conventional pigment making visual diagnosis difficult.

Appearance: May seem pink or red similar to other skin disorders; a biopsy is required for confirmation.

STAGES AND PROGRESSION

Melanoma is divided into stages based on how far it has progressed with each stage representing a different degree of progression. The staging system aids in treatment planning and prognosis.

Stage 0 (In Situ Melanoma):

Characteristics: Restricted to the skin's top layer. Progression: Epidermis-only with no invasion into deeper layers. Surgical removal has a high cure rate.

Stage One:

Melanoma that is localized and has thin tumors. Progression is limited to the skin with some little invasion into the dermis. With surgical intervention, the prognosis is favorable.

Stage 2:

Melanoma that is localized and has thicker tumours.Tumour growth may spread deeper into the skin as it progresses. The primary treatment remains surgical excision and the risk of spread increases with tumor thickness.

Stage Three:

Melanoma that has spread to the lymph nodes in the region.Lymph node involvement suggests a greater risk of metastasis. Surgical lymph node excision, immunotherapy or targeted therapy are frequently used in treatment.

Stage 4:

Melanoma that has spread to other parts of the body.Progression: The cancer spreads to distant organs such as the lungs, liver, brain or other locations. Systemic therapies such as immunotherapy or targeted therapy are used in treatment.

CHAPTER 2: NUTRITIONAL GUIDELINES FOR MELANOMA

1. Foods High in Antioxidants:

   The goal is to combat oxidative stress. Berries, citrus fruits, leafy greens and nuts are among examples.

2. Fatty Acids Omega-3:

   The goal is to control inflammation.Fatty fish (salmon, mackerel) chia seeds, flaxseeds and walnuts are good sources.

3. C and E vitamins:

   Goal: To promote skin health and healing.Citrus fruits, bell peppers, almonds and sunflower seeds are all good sources.

4. Ginger with turmeric:

   Natural anti-inflammatory qualities are used. In cooking use fresh or ground turmeric and ginger.

5. Tea, Green:

   Polyphenols having anti-cancer effects are found in this product. Recommendation: Use in beverages or cooking.

6. Vegetables in a Variety of Colors:

   Provide a variety of nutrients. Carrots, sweet potatoes and bell peppers are some examples.

7. Proteins that are low in fat:

   Supporting muscle strength during treatment.Skinless poultry, fish, lentils and tofu are also good sources.

8. Hydration:

   Maintain general health and aid with rehabilitation.Recommendation: Drink plenty of water every day.

9. Limit your intake of processed foods:

   Reduce your intake of additives and preservatives. Advice: When feasible, choose complete unprocessed meals.

IMPACT OF DIET ON MELANOMA

1. **Prevention:**

   A diet high in antioxidants and nutrients may help reduce the incidence of melanoma by countering oxidative stress and improving general skin health. Recommendation: Focus on a colorful plant-based diet rich in fruits, vegetables and foods high in vitamins C and E.

2. Immune Boost:

   Nutrient-dense diets reinforce the immune system, assisting the body in identifying and eliminating aberrant cells, including melanoma cells. To assist the body's defense mechanisms, include lean proteins, omega-3 fatty acids and immune-boosting foods.

3. Inflammation Control:

   Chronic inflammation has been related to cancer progression and specific dietary choices can aid in inflammation management. Recommendation: Include anti-inflammatory foods like turmeric, ginger and omega-3-rich sources in your diet to produce an environment that is less conducive to the growth of melanoma.

4. Skin Care:

   Nutrition has a direct impact on skin integrity and resilience to UV-induced damage which is a key risk factor for melanoma. Consume meals high in vitamins C and E to promote skin regeneration and protection.

5. Treatment Assistance:

   Role: Proper nutrition can help with melanoma treatment side effects and overall well-being during the healing process.Individualised dietary programmes including water and nutrient-dense alternatives can help to alleviate treatment-related complications.

6. Holistic Health:

   Beyond specific nutrients, a well-balanced diet promotes general health, encouraging strength and perseverance in the face of melanoma.

Recommendation: Eat a well-balanced varied diet rich in healthy foods and drink enough water.

FOODS WITH ANTI-INFLAMMATORY PROPERTIES

1. Fish with a lot of fat:

   Salmon, mackerel, sardines and trout are among examples. Omega-3 fatty acids are anti-inflammatory components.

2. Berries:

   Blueberries, strawberries, raspberries and blackberries are some examples. Anthocyanins and quercetin are anti-inflammatory components.

3. Broccoli:

   Sulforaphane and kaempferol are anti-inflammatory ingredients.

4. Avocado:

   Monounsaturated fats and antioxidants are anti-inflammatory components.

5. Turmeric:

   Curcumin is the active ingredient. Anti-Inflammatory Effects: Strong anti-inflammatory and antioxidant properties.

6. Tea, Green:

   Catechins, notably epigallocatechin gallate (EGCG) are anti-inflammatory components.

7. Chocolate, dark:

   Caution: Only in moderation with a high cocoa content (70% or above). Flavanols are anti-inflammatory components.

8. Tomatoes:

   Lycopene, vitamin C and beta-carotene are anti-inflammatory components.

9. Extra Virgin Olive Oil:

   Oleocanthal and oleic acid are anti-inflammatory components.

10. Chia Seeds, Walnut Ginger.

    Omega-3 fatty acids and alpha-linolenic acid are anti-inflammatory components.

IMPORTANCE OF HYDRATION

1. Molecular Function:
   Water is necessary for cellular functions because it facilitates nutrition transport, temperature regulation and overall cellular function.
2. Detoxification:
   Water helps the kidneys filter and eliminate toxins from the body, providing a healthy and effective detoxification process.
3. Temperature Control:
   Water regulates body temperature through sweating and evaporative cooling, which is important for avoiding overheating during physical exercise or in hot surroundings.
4. Lubrication of joints:
   Role: Proper hydration keeps joints lubricated, minimizing friction and promoting smooth movement.
5. Digestive Wellness:
   Water aids in nutrition digestion and absorption, avoiding constipation and promoting overall gastrointestinal health.
6. Cognitive Ability:
   Dehydration has the potential to impair cognitive function, particularly focus and attentiveness. Keeping hydrated is essential for peak mental efficiency.
7. Skin Care:
   Skin that is well-hydrated appears more vivid and supple. Water promotes skin suppleness and aids the body's natural processes of skin cell repair and rejuvenation.
8. Levels of Energy:
   Dehydration can cause fatigue and a reduction in energy levels. Maintaining physical and mental energy requires staying hydrated.
9. Exercise Efficiency:
   Proper hydration is essential for athletes and individuals participating in physical activities since it aids in endurance, strength and overall performance.
10. Metabolic Functions:
    Water has a role in several metabolic events in the body, including the breakdown of foods for energy.
11. Dehydration-Related Complications Prevention:
    Adequate hydration is critical to avoiding dehydration-related consequences such as heat-related diseases, kidney stones and urinary tract infections.

CHAPTER 3: FRIENDLY BREAKFAST OPTION

Berry Smoothie Bowl:

Ingredients:

- 1 cup mixed berries (blueberries, strawberries, raspberries)
- 1/2 ripe banana
- 1/2 cup spinach leaves
- 1/4 cup Greek yogurt (unsweetened)
- 1 tablespoon chia seeds
- 1/2 cup almond milk (unsweetened)
- 1 teaspoon honey (optional, for sweetness)
- 1/4 cup walnuts or flaxseeds (optional, for added nutrients)

Instructions:

1. Prepare the Berries: Wash the berries thoroughly and slice the strawberries if needed.
2. Blend the Base: In a blender, combine the mixed berries, ripe banana, spinach leaves, Greek yogurt, chia seeds, and almond milk.
3. Blend Until Smooth: Blend the ingredients until you achieve a smooth and creamy consistency.
4. Taste and Sweeten: Taste the mixture and add honey if desired. Blend again to incorporate the sweetness.
5. Pour into a Bowl: Transfer the smoothie into a bowl, ensuring a smooth and even layer.
6. Top with Nutrients: Sprinkle the smoothie bowl with additional nutrients by adding walnuts or flaxseeds.

Salmon and Avocado Toast:

Ingredients:

- 2 slices whole-grain bread

- 1 ripe avocado
- 150g smoked salmon
- 1 tablespoon lemon juice
- Salt and pepper to taste
- Optional toppings: cherry tomatoes, microgreens, or red onion slices

Instructions:

1. Toast the Bread: Toast the whole-grain bread slices to your desired level of crispiness.
2. Prepare the Avocado: Mash the ripe avocado in a bowl and add lemon juice, salt, and pepper. Mix well to create a smooth avocado spread.
3. Spread Avocado: Evenly spread the mashed avocado over the toasted bread slices.
4. Add Smoked Salmon: Lay the smoked salmon on top of the avocado spread, covering the entire surface of the bread.
5. Season to Taste: Sprinkle a bit of salt and pepper over the smoked salmon to taste.
6. Optional Toppings: Enhance the toast by adding optional toppings like cherry tomatoes, microgreens, or thinly sliced red onions for added flavor and freshness.
7. Serve and Enjoy: Your delicious Salmon and Avocado Toast is ready to be served. It makes for a nutritious and satisfying meal, rich in omega-3 fatty acids and other essential nutrients.

Turmeric Scrambled Eggs:

Ingredients:

- 4 large eggs
- 1/2 teaspoon ground turmeric
- 1 tablespoon milk (optional)
- Salt and pepper to taste
- 1 tablespoon olive oil or butter
- Fresh herbs (chopped parsley or cilantro, for garnish)

Instructions:

1. Crack and Beat Eggs: Crack the eggs into a bowl and beat them until the yolks and whites are well combined.

2. Add Turmeric: Sprinkle ground turmeric over the beaten eggs. If you like, add a tablespoon of milk for fluffier eggs. Mix well to ensure the turmeric is evenly distributed.

3. Season with Salt and Pepper: Season the egg mixture with salt and pepper to taste. Mix again.

4. Heat Oil or Butter: In a non-stick skillet, heat olive oil or butter over medium heat until melted and hot.

5. Scramble Eggs: Pour the turmeric-infused egg mixture into the skillet. Allow the eggs to set for a moment before gently stirring with a spatula. Continue stirring occasionally until the eggs are cooked to your desired consistency.

6. Garnish: Just before removing from heat, sprinkle fresh herbs like chopped parsley or cilantro over the scrambled eggs for added flavor and freshness.

7. Serve Immediately: Transfer the turmeric scrambled eggs to a plate and serve hot. You can pair them with whole-grain toast, avocado, or your favorite sides.

Chia Seed Pudding with Berries:

Ingredients:

- 1/4 cup chia seeds
- 1 cup almond milk (or any milk of your choice)
- 1 tablespoon honey or maple syrup (optional, for sweetness)
- 1/2 teaspoon vanilla extract
- Mixed berries (strawberries, blueberries, raspberries) for topping
- Nuts or shredded coconut for garnish (optional)

Instructions:

1. Mix Chia Seeds and Liquid: In a bowl, combine chia seeds and almond milk. Stir well to ensure the chia seeds are evenly distributed.

2. Add Sweetener and Vanilla: If desired, add honey or maple syrup for sweetness and vanilla extract for flavor. Mix thoroughly.

3. Let it Set: Cover the bowl and refrigerate the mixture for at least 2-3 hours, or preferably overnight. This allows the chia seeds to absorb the liquid and create a pudding-like consistency.

4. Stir Before Serving: After the chia pudding has set, give it a good stir to break up any clumps and ensure a smooth texture.

5. Layer with Berries: In serving glasses or bowls, layer the chia pudding with mixed berries. You can also alternate layers for a visually appealing presentation.

6. Garnish: Top the chia seed pudding with additional berries and, if desired, garnish with nuts or shredded coconut for added texture.

7. Serve and Enjoy: Your delicious and nutritious Chia Seed Pudding with Berries is ready to be enjoyed as a healthy breakfast or snack.

Quinoa Breakfast Bowl:

Ingredients:

- 1/2 cup quinoa, rinsed
- 1 cup almond milk (or any milk of your choice)
- 1 tablespoon honey or maple syrup
- 1/2 teaspoon vanilla extract
- Fresh fruits (berries, sliced banana, kiwi)
- Nuts and seeds (almonds, chia seeds, pumpkin seeds)
- Greek yogurt or plant-based yogurt
- Optional: cinnamon or nutmeg for extra flavor

Instructions:

1. Cook Quinoa: In a saucepan, combine quinoa and almond milk. Bring to a boil, then reduce heat to low, cover, and simmer for 15-20 minutes or until the quinoa is cooked and has absorbed the liquid.

2. Sweeten and Flavor: Once quinoa is cooked, stir in honey or maple syrup and vanilla extract. Mix well to evenly distribute sweetness and flavor.

3. Prepare Toppings: While quinoa is cooking, chop fresh fruits and gather nuts and seeds for toppings.

4. Assemble Breakfast Bowl: Spoon the sweetened quinoa into a bowl. Top with a generous portion of fresh fruits, a dollop of Greek yogurt, and a sprinkle of nuts and seeds.

5. Add Extra Flavor (Optional): If desired, dust the bowl with a pinch of cinnamon or nutmeg for added warmth and depth of flavor.

6. Serve and Enjoy: Your nutritious and satisfying Quinoa Breakfast Bowl is ready to be enjoyed. Customize the toppings based on your preferences and dietary needs.

Green Tea Oatmeal:

Ingredients:

- 1 cup rolled oats
- 2 cups water
- 1 green tea bag (or 1 teaspoon loose green tea leaves)
- 1 tablespoon honey or maple syrup
- 1/2 teaspoon matcha powder
- Fresh fruit slices (e.g., kiwi, strawberries) for topping
- Nuts or seeds (e.g., almonds, chia seeds) for garnish

Instructions:

1. Brew Green Tea: Heat 2 cups of water until just before boiling. Steep the green tea bag (or loose green tea leaves) in the hot water for 3-5 minutes. Remove the tea bag or strain the leaves, and set aside the brewed green tea.

2. Cook Oats: In a saucepan, combine rolled oats with the brewed green tea. Cook over medium heat, stirring occasionally, until the oats have absorbed most of the liquid and reached your desired consistency.

3. Sweeten with Honey and Add Matcha: Stir in honey or maple syrup for sweetness. Add matcha powder to the oatmeal, mixing well to incorporate the vibrant green tea flavor.

4. Top with Fresh Fruit: Once the oatmeal is cooked, transfer it to a bowl. Top with fresh fruit slices, such as kiwi and strawberries, for a burst of color and additional vitamins.

5. Garnish with Nuts or Seeds: Sprinkle your choice of nuts or seeds, like almonds or chia seeds, over the oatmeal for added texture and nutritional benefits.

6. Serve Warm: Your Green Tea Oatmeal is ready to be served. Enjoy it warm for a comforting and nutritious breakfast.

Walnut and Banana Pancakes:

Ingredients:

- 1 cup all-purpose flour
- 2 tablespoons sugar
- 1 teaspoon baking powder
- 1/2 teaspoon baking soda
- 1/4 teaspoon salt
- 1 cup buttermilk
- 1 large egg
- 2 ripe bananas, mashed
- 1/2 cup chopped walnuts
- 1 teaspoon vanilla extract
- Butter or oil for cooking

Instructions:

1. Mix Dry Ingredients: In a large bowl, whisk together the flour, sugar, baking powder, baking soda, and salt.

2. Combine Wet Ingredients: In a separate bowl, beat the egg and then add buttermilk, mashed bananas, chopped walnuts, and vanilla extract. Mix until well combined.

3. Combine Wet and Dry Ingredients: Pour the wet ingredients into the dry ingredients. Stir until just combined. The batter may be a bit lumpy, which is okay. Do not overmix.

4. Heat Griddle or Pan: Heat a griddle or non-stick pan over medium heat. Add a small amount of butter or oil to coat the surface.

5. Cook Pancakes: Pour 1/4 cup portions of batter onto the griddle. Cook until bubbles form on the surface, then flip and cook the other side until golden brown.

6. Keep Warm: Transfer the cooked pancakes to a plate and keep them warm in a low-temperature oven while you cook the remaining batter.

7. Serve: Serve the Walnut and Banana Pancakes warm. Top with additional sliced bananas, a sprinkle of chopped walnuts, and a drizzle of maple syrup if desired.

Tomato and Basil Frittata:

Ingredients:

- 6 large eggs
- 1 cup cherry tomatoes, halved
- 1/4 cup fresh basil, chopped
- 1/2 cup feta cheese, crumbled
- 1/4 cup grated Parmesan cheese
- 1/2 teaspoon salt
- 1/4 teaspoon black pepper
- 2 tablespoons olive oil
- Optional: Red pepper flakes for added spice

Instructions:

1. Preheat Oven: Preheat your oven broiler.

2. Whisk Eggs: In a bowl, whisk the eggs until well beaten. Add salt, black pepper, and chopped basil. Whisk to combine.

3. Prepare Tomatoes: Heat olive oil in an oven-safe skillet over medium heat. Add halved cherry tomatoes to the skillet and cook for 2-3 minutes until they start to soften.

4. Pour Egg Mixture: Pour the whisked egg mixture over the tomatoes in the skillet. Allow the edges to set for a minute.

5. Add Cheeses: Sprinkle crumbled feta and grated Parmesan evenly over the egg mixture.

6. Cook on Stovetop: Cook on the stovetop for 3-5 minutes or until the edges start to set.

7. Broil in Oven: Transfer the skillet to the preheated oven and broil for 3-4 minutes or until the frittata is set in the center and the top is lightly browned.

8. Optional Spice: If desired, sprinkle red pepper flakes over the frittata for a bit of spice.

9. Serve Warm: Carefully remove the skillet from the oven. Allow the frittata to cool for a moment, then slice and serve warm.

Almond Butter and Berry Wrap:

Ingredients:
- 1 whole-grain or multigrain wrap
- 2 tablespoons almond butter (unsweetened)
- 1/2 cup mixed berries (strawberries, blueberries, raspberries)
- 1 teaspoon honey or maple syrup (optional, for extra sweetness)
- Chia seeds or sliced almonds for added crunch (optional)

Instructions:
1. Prepare the Wrap: Lay the whole-grain or multigrain wrap on a clean surface.
2. Spread Almond Butter: Evenly spread almond butter over the entire surface of the wrap.
3. Add Mixed Berries: Scatter mixed berries across the center of the wrap. You can mix and match berries for a variety of flavors.

4. Drizzle with Sweetener (Optional): If you desire additional sweetness, drizzle honey or maple syrup over the berries.
5. Sprinkle with Crunchy Toppings (Optional): For added texture, sprinkle chia seeds or sliced almonds over the berries.
6. Fold and Roll: Carefully fold the sides of the wrap and then roll it from the bottom, creating a snug wrap.
7. Slice and Serve: Use a sharp knife to slice the wrap in half diagonally. This makes it easier to handle and enjoy.
8. Serve Immediately: Your Almond Butter and Berry Wrap is ready to be enjoyed. Serve it immediately for the best texture and flavor.

Spinach and Mushroom Omelette:

Ingredients:

- 3 large eggs
- 1/2 cup fresh spinach, chopped
- 1/2 cup mushrooms, sliced
- 1/4 cup onion, finely diced
- 1/4 cup shredded cheese (your choice, like cheddar or feta)
- Salt and pepper to taste
- 1 tablespoon olive oil or butter
- Fresh herbs (optional, for garnish)

Instructions:

1. Prepare Ingredients: Chop the fresh spinach, slice the mushrooms, and finely dice the onion.
2. Sauté Vegetables: In a non-stick skillet, heat olive oil or butter over medium heat. Sauté the mushrooms and onions until they are softened and the mushrooms release their moisture.
3. Add Spinach: Add the chopped spinach to the skillet and cook until wilted. Season with salt and pepper to taste. Set aside the sautéed vegetables.
4. Whisk Eggs: In a bowl, whisk the eggs until well beaten. Season with a pinch of salt and pepper.
5. Cook Eggs: Heat the skillet over medium-low heat. Pour the beaten eggs into the skillet, tilting it to spread the eggs evenly.
6. Add Vegetables and Cheese: Once the edges of the omelet start to set, add the sautéed vegetables evenly over one half of the omelet. Sprinkle shredded cheese on top.

7. Fold and Cook: Carefully fold the other half of the omelet over the vegetables and cheese. Cook for an additional minute or until the cheese is melted and the omelet is cooked to your liking.

8. Garnish and Serve: Slide the omelet onto a plate, garnish with fresh herbs if desired, and serve hot.

Mango and Turmeric Smoothie:

Ingredients:
- 1 cup frozen mango chunks
- 1/2 cup plain Greek yogurt
- 1/2 cup almond milk (or any milk of your choice)
- 1/2 teaspoon ground turmeric
- 1 tablespoon honey or maple syrup (optional, for sweetness)
- 1/2 teaspoon fresh ginger, grated (optional)
- Ice cubes (optional)
- Chia seeds or flax seeds for garnish (optional)

Instructions:
1. Prepare Ingredients: Ensure the frozen mango chunks are ready. If using fresh mango, you can add ice cubes to the blender for a chilled smoothie.
2. Add Mango to Blender: Place the frozen mango chunks into a blender.
3. Combine Ingredients: Add Greek yogurt, almond milk, ground turmeric, and grated ginger to the blender.
4. Sweeten (Optional): If you prefer a sweeter smoothie, add honey or maple syrup. Adjust the sweetness to your liking.
5. Blend Until Smooth: Blend the ingredients until you achieve a smooth and creamy consistency.
6. Taste and Adjust: Taste the smoothie and adjust the sweetness or turmeric level if necessary.
7. Serve in a Glass: Pour the Mango and Turmeric Smoothie into a glass.
8. Garnish (Optional): Sprinkle chia seeds or flaxseeds on top for added texture and nutritional benefits.
9. Serve and Enjoy: Your vibrant and refreshing Mango and Turmeric Smoothie is ready to be enjoyed. It's a delicious way to incorporate the health benefits of turmeric into your diet.

Salmon and Kale Salad:

Ingredients:

For the Salmon:

- 2 salmon fillets
- 1 tablespoon olive oil
- Salt and pepper to taste
- 1 teaspoon lemon zest
- 1 tablespoon lemon juice

For the Salad:

- 4 cups kale, stems removed and leaves chopped
- 1 cup cherry tomatoes, halved
- 1/2 cucumber, sliced
- 1/4 red onion, thinly sliced
- 1/4 cup feta cheese, crumbled
- 1/4 cup walnuts, chopped (optional)

For the Dressing:

- 3 tablespoons olive oil
- 1 tablespoon balsamic vinegar
- 1 teaspoon Dijon mustard
- 1 clove garlic, minced
- Salt and pepper to taste

Instructions:

Prepare the Salmon:

1. Preheat the oven to 400°F (200°C).
2. Rub salmon fillets with olive oil, salt, and pepper. Place them on a baking sheet.
3. Sprinkle lemon zest over the salmon and drizzle with lemon juice.

4. Bake for 12-15 minutes or until the salmon is cooked through and flakes easily with a fork.

5. Remove from the oven and let it rest for a few minutes. Once cooled slightly, flake the salmon into bite-sized pieces.

Prepare the Salad:

1. In a large salad bowl, combine chopped kale, cherry tomatoes, cucumber, red onion, feta cheese, and walnuts (if using).

2. Add the flaked salmon on top.

Prepare the Dressing:

1. In a small bowl, whisk together olive oil, balsamic vinegar, Dijon mustard, minced garlic, salt, and pepper.

2. Pour the dressing over the salad and toss until all ingredients are well coated.

3. Allow the salad to sit for a few minutes to let the flavors meld.

4. Serve immediately, and enjoy your nutritious Salmon and Kale Salad!

Quinoa and Chickpea Bowl:

Ingredients:

For the Quinoa and Chickpeas:

- 1 cup quinoa, rinsed
- 2 cups water or vegetable broth
- 1 can (15 oz) chickpeas, drained and rinsed
- 1 tablespoon olive oil
- 1 teaspoon ground cumin
- 1 teaspoon paprika
- Salt and pepper to taste

For the Bowl:

- 2 cups mixed greens (spinach, kale, arugula, etc.)
- 1 cup cherry tomatoes, halved
- 1 cucumber, diced

- 1/2 red onion, finely chopped
- 1/4 cup feta cheese, crumbled (optional)

For the Dressing:

- 3 tablespoons olive oil
- 1 tablespoon balsamic vinegar
- 1 clove garlic, minced
- 1 teaspoon honey or maple syrup
- Salt and pepper to taste

Instructions:

Prepare Quinoa and Chickpeas:

1. In a medium saucepan, combine quinoa and water (or vegetable broth). Bring to a boil, then reduce heat to low, cover, and simmer for 15-20 minutes or until quinoa is cooked and water is absorbed.
2. In a skillet, heat olive oil over medium heat. Add chickpeas, cumin, paprika, salt, and pepper. Sauté for 5-7 minutes until chickpeas are lightly browned and coated with spices.
3. Combine cooked quinoa and chickpeas in a bowl.

Prepare the Bowl:

1. In serving bowls, arrange a bed of mixed greens.
2. Top the greens with the quinoa and chickpea mixture.
3. Add cherry tomatoes, diced cucumber, chopped red onion, and crumbled feta cheese (if using).

Prepare the Dressing:

1. In a small bowl, whisk together olive oil, balsamic vinegar, minced garlic, honey (or maple syrup), salt, and pepper.
2. Drizzle the dressing over the quinoa and vegetable mixture.
3. Toss the ingredients gently to coat everything with the dressing.
4. Serve immediately, and enjoy your wholesome Quinoa and Chickpea Bowl!

Turkey and Avocado Wrap with Spinach:

Ingredients:

- 1 large whole-grain or spinach tortilla
- 4 oz sliced turkey breast
- 1/2 avocado, sliced
- 1 cup fresh spinach leaves
- 1/4 cup cherry tomatoes, halved
- 1/4 cup red onion, thinly sliced
- 1 tablespoon mayonnaise or Greek yogurt
- 1 teaspoon Dijon mustard
- Salt and pepper to taste

Instructions:

1. Prepare Ingredients: Slice the turkey breast, avocado, cherry tomatoes, and red onion.
2. Warm the Tortilla: If desired, briefly warm the tortilla in a dry skillet or microwave for a few seconds to make it more pliable.
3. Spread Sauce: In the center of the tortilla, spread mayonnaise or Greek yogurt. Drizzle Dijon mustard over the sauce.
4. Layer Ingredients: Arrange the sliced turkey on top of the sauce. Add avocado slices, fresh spinach leaves, halved cherry tomatoes, and thinly sliced red onion.
5. Season with Salt and Pepper: Sprinkle salt and pepper over the ingredients to taste.
6. Wrap It Up: Fold the sides of the tortilla towards the center and then roll it from the bottom, creating a tight wrap.
7. Slice and Serve: Carefully slice the wrap in half diagonally for easier handling.
8. Serve Immediately: Your Turkey and Avocado Wrap with Spinach is ready to be enjoyed. Serve it immediately for the best texture and flavor.

Tomato and Basil Lentil Soup:

Ingredients:

- 1 cup dried green or brown lentils, rinsed
- 1 can (14 oz) diced tomatoes
- 1 large onion, diced
- 2 carrots, diced
- 2 celery stalks, diced
- 3 cloves garlic, minced
- 1 teaspoon dried oregano
- 1 teaspoon dried thyme
- 1 bay leaf
- 4 cups vegetable broth
- 2 cups water
- Salt and pepper to taste
- 1 cup fresh basil leaves, chopped
- 2 tablespoons olive oil
- Grated Parmesan cheese for garnish (optional)

Instructions:

1. Prepare Lentils: Rinse the lentils under cold water and set aside.
2. Sauté Vegetables: In a large pot, heat olive oil over medium heat. Add diced onion, carrots, and celery. Sauté until vegetables are softened, about 5-7 minutes.
3. Add Garlic and Herbs: Stir in minced garlic, dried oregano, dried thyme, and the bay leaf. Cook for an additional 1-2 minutes until fragrant.
4. Add Lentils and Tomatoes: Add rinsed lentils and canned diced tomatoes (with their juice) to the pot. Stir to combine with the sautéed vegetables.
5. Pour in Broth and Water: Pour in the vegetable broth and water. Season with salt and pepper to taste.
6. Simmer: Bring the soup to a boil, then reduce the heat to low, cover, and let it simmer for about 25-30 minutes or until lentils are tender.
7. Add Fresh Basil: Stir in the chopped fresh basil. Simmer for an additional 5 minutes to allow the flavors to meld.

8. Adjust Seasoning: Taste the soup and adjust the seasoning if necessary. Remove the bay leaf.
9. Serve: Ladle the Tomato and Basil Lentil Soup into bowls. Optionally, garnish with grated Parmesan cheese.
10. Enjoy: Serve hot and enjoy your comforting and nutritious Tomato and Basil Lentil Soup.

Grilled Chicken and Quinoa Stuffed Bell Peppers

Ingredients:

- 4 large bell peppers (any color)
- 1 cup quinoa, cooked
- 1 lb boneless, skinless chicken breasts
- 1 tablespoon olive oil
- 1 onion, finely chopped
- 2 cloves garlic, minced
- 1 teaspoon ground cumin
- 1 teaspoon smoked paprika
- Salt and pepper to taste
- 1 can (14 oz) black beans, drained and rinsed
- 1 cup corn kernels (fresh or frozen)
- 1 cup cherry tomatoes, halved
- 1 cup shredded cheese (cheddar, Monterey Jack, or a blend)
- Fresh cilantro or parsley for garnish (optional)
- Lime wedges for serving

Instructions:

1. Preheat Grill: Preheat your grill to medium-high heat.
2. Prepare Bell Peppers: Cut the bell peppers in half lengthwise, removing the seeds and membranes. Lightly brush the outside of the peppers with olive oil.

3. Grill Chicken: Season chicken breasts with cumin, smoked paprika, salt, and pepper. Grill the chicken for 6-8 minutes per side or until fully cooked. Allow it to rest for a few minutes, then dice into small pieces.

4. Sauté Onion and Garlic: In a skillet, heat olive oil over medium heat. Add chopped onion and sauté until translucent. Add minced garlic and cook for an additional 1-2 minutes.

5. Combine Ingredients: In a large bowl, combine cooked quinoa, diced grilled chicken, sautéed onion and garlic, black beans, corn, cherry tomatoes, and half of the shredded cheese. Mix well.

6. Stuff Bell Peppers: Stuff each bell pepper half with the quinoa and chicken mixture. Press down gently to pack the filling.

7. Grill Stuffed Peppers: Place the stuffed peppers on the preheated grill. Close the lid and grill for 10-15 minutes or until the peppers are tender and the filling is heated through.

8. Add Cheese and Melt: Sprinkle the remaining shredded cheese over the stuffed peppers. Close the grill lid and let the cheese melt for 2-3 minutes.

9. Garnish and Serve: Remove the stuffed peppers from the grill. Garnish with fresh cilantro or parsley if desired. Serve with lime wedges on the side.

10. Enjoy: These Grilled Chicken and Quinoa Stuffed Bell Peppers are ready to be enjoyed as a flavorful and nutritious meal.

Mango and Avocado Chicken Salad:

Ingredients:

For the Salad:

- 2 boneless, skinless chicken breasts
- Salt and pepper to taste
- 1 tablespoon olive oil
- 6 cups mixed salad greens (e.g., spinach, arugula, romaine)
- 1 ripe mango, peeled, pitted, and diced

- 1 ripe avocado, peeled, pitted, and sliced
- 1/4 red onion, thinly sliced
- 1/4 cup chopped fresh cilantro or mint

For the Dressing:

- 3 tablespoons olive oil
- 2 tablespoons lime juice
- 1 tablespoon honey
- 1 teaspoon Dijon mustard
- Salt and pepper to taste

Instructions:

1. Prepare Chicken: Season chicken breasts with salt and pepper. In a skillet over medium-high heat, heat olive oil. Cook the chicken for about 6-7 minutes per side or until fully cooked. Allow it to rest for a few minutes, then slice into thin strips.
2. Prepare Salad Ingredients: In a large salad bowl, combine the mixed greens, diced mango, sliced avocado, red onion, and chopped cilantro or mint.
3. Make the Dressing: In a small bowl, whisk together olive oil, lime juice, honey, Dijon mustard, salt, and pepper.
4. Combine Salad and Chicken: Add the sliced chicken to the salad bowl.
5. Drizzle with Dressing: Pour the dressing over the salad and chicken. Toss gently to coat all ingredients with the dressing.
6. Serve: Plate the Mango and Avocado Chicken Salad on individual serving plates or a large platter.
7. Garnish (Optional): Garnish with additional cilantro or mint if desired.
8. Enjoy: Your refreshing and flavorful Mango and Avocado Chicken Salad is ready to be enjoyed as a light and satisfying meal.

Tuna and White Bean Salad:

Ingredients:

- 2 cans (about 12 oz each) white beans (cannellini or navy), drained and rinsed

- 2 cans (about 5 oz each) tuna in water, drained
- 1/2 red onion, finely chopped
- 1 cup cherry tomatoes, halved
- 1/4 cup Kalamata olives, pitted and sliced
- 1/4 cup fresh parsley, chopped
- 2 tablespoons capers, drained
- 2 tablespoons red wine vinegar
- 3 tablespoons extra-virgin olive oil
- Salt and pepper to taste
- 1 lemon, sliced for garnish (optional)

Instructions:

1. Prepare White Beans: In a large bowl, combine the drained and rinsed white beans.
2. Add Tuna: Flake the drained tuna into the bowl with the white beans.
3. Add Vegetables and Herbs: Add chopped red onion, halved cherry tomatoes, sliced Kalamata olives, chopped fresh parsley, and capers to the bowl.
4. Make the Dressing: In a small bowl, whisk together red wine vinegar, extra-virgin olive oil, salt, and pepper.
5. Combine and Toss: Pour the dressing over the bean and tuna mixture. Gently toss the ingredients until everything is well coated.
6. Adjust Seasoning: Taste the salad and adjust the seasoning if needed.
7. Chill (Optional): For enhanced flavor, cover the bowl and let the salad chill in the refrigerator for at least 30 minutes before serving.
8. Serve: Portion the Tuna and White Bean Salad onto plates. Optionally, garnish with lemon slices.
9. Enjoy: Your light, protein-packed Tuna and White Bean Salad is ready to be enjoyed as a nutritious and satisfying meal.

Broccoli and Almond Quinoa Bowl:

Ingredients:

- 1 cup quinoa, rinsed
- 2 cups broccoli florets
- 1/3 cup almonds, sliced or chopped
- 1 tablespoon olive oil
- 2 cloves garlic, minced
- 1 teaspoon lemon zest
- 2 tablespoons lemon juice
- Salt and pepper to taste
- 1/4 cup fresh parsley, chopped (optional, for garnish)

Instructions:

1. Prepare Quinoa: In a medium saucepan, combine quinoa with 2 cups of water. Bring to a boil, then reduce heat to low, cover, and simmer for 15-20 minutes or until quinoa is cooked and water is absorbed.

2. Steam Broccoli: While the quinoa is cooking, steam the broccoli until it's tender but still has a slight crunch. You can steam it on the stovetop or use a microwave-safe bowl with a bit of water, covered with a microwave-safe plate.

3. Toast Almonds: In a dry skillet over medium heat, toast the almonds until they become golden and fragrant. Stir frequently to prevent burning. Set aside.

4. Sauté Garlic: In the same skillet, heat olive oil over medium heat. Add minced garlic and sauté for about 1-2 minutes until it becomes fragrant.

5. Combine Quinoa, Broccoli, and Almonds: Add the cooked quinoa, steamed broccoli, and toasted almonds to the skillet with the sautéed garlic. Toss the ingredients together.

6. Add Lemon Zest and Juice: Sprinkle lemon zest and drizzle lemon juice over the quinoa mixture. Toss again to evenly distribute the flavors.

7. Season with Salt and Pepper: Season with salt and pepper to taste. Adjust the seasoning as needed.

8. Garnish (Optional): If desired, garnish the Broccoli and Almond Quinoa Bowl with chopped fresh parsley for added freshness.

9. Serve Warm: Portion the quinoa bowl into serving dishes and serve warm.

10. Enjoy: Your nutritious and flavorful Broccoli and Almond Quinoa Bowl is ready to be enjoyed as a wholesome meal.

Shrimp and Vegetable Stir-Fry:

Ingredients:

- 1 lb large shrimp, peeled and deveined
- 2 cups broccoli florets
- 1 bell pepper, thinly sliced (any color)
- 1 carrot, julienned
- 1 cup snap peas, ends trimmed
- 3 cloves garlic, minced
- 1 tablespoon fresh ginger, grated
- 3 tablespoons soy sauce
- 1 tablespoon oyster sauce
- 1 tablespoon cornstarch
- 2 tablespoons water
- 2 tablespoons sesame oil
- 2 tablespoons vegetable oil (for cooking)
- Cooked rice or noodles for serving

Instructions:

1. Prepare Shrimp: Pat the shrimp dry with a paper towel. In a bowl, mix the shrimp with 1 tablespoon of soy sauce and set aside.

2. Mix Sauce: In a small bowl, whisk together the remaining soy sauce, oyster sauce, cornstarch, and water. Set aside.

3. Heat Wok or Skillet: Heat vegetable oil in a wok or large skillet over medium-high heat.

4. Sauté Shrimp: Add the shrimp to the hot pan and stir-fry for 2-3 minutes or until they turn pink and opaque. Remove the shrimp from the pan and set aside.

5. Stir-Fry Vegetables: In the same pan, add a bit more oil if needed. Add garlic and ginger, sauté for about 30 seconds until fragrant. Add broccoli, bell pepper, carrot, and snap peas. Stir-fry for 3-4 minutes or until vegetables are crisp-tender.

6. Combine Shrimp and Vegetables: Return the cooked shrimp to the pan with the vegetables. Toss everything together.

7. Pour Sauce: Pour the sauce over the shrimp and vegetables. Stir well to coat everything evenly. Cook for an additional 1-2 minutes until the sauce thickens.

8. Drizzle with Sesame Oil: Drizzle sesame oil over the stir-fry and toss to combine.

9. Serve: Serve the Shrimp and Vegetable Stir-Fry over cooked rice or noodles.

10. Enjoy: Your quick and delicious Shrimp and Vegetable Stir-Fry is ready to be enjoyed as a flavorful and nutritious meal.

Eggplant and Chickpea Curry:

Ingredients:

- 1 large eggplant, cut into cubes
- 1 can (15 oz) chickpeas, drained and rinsed
- 1 large onion, finely chopped
- 3 cloves garlic, minced
- 1 tablespoon fresh ginger, grated
- 1 can (14 oz) diced tomatoes
- 1 can (14 oz) coconut milk
- 2 tablespoons curry powder
- 1 teaspoon ground cumin
- 1 teaspoon ground coriander
- 1/2 teaspoon turmeric
- 1/2 teaspoon cayenne pepper (adjust to taste)
- Salt and pepper to taste

- 2 tablespoons vegetable oil

- Fresh cilantro for garnish

- Cooked rice or naan for serving

Instructions:

1. Prep Ingredients: Cut the eggplant into cubes, chop the onion, mince the garlic, and grate the fresh ginger.
2. Sauté Onion, Garlic, and Ginger: In a large pan or pot, heat vegetable oil over medium heat. Add chopped onion and sauté until softened. Add minced garlic and grated ginger, sauté for an additional 1-2 minutes until fragrant.
3. Add Spices: Stir in curry powder, ground cumin, ground coriander, turmeric, and cayenne pepper. Cook for 1-2 minutes to toast the spices.
4. Add Eggplant and Chickpeas: Add the eggplant cubes and chickpeas to the pan. Stir to coat them with the spices.
5. Pour in Diced Tomatoes and Coconut Milk: Add diced tomatoes (with their juice) and coconut milk to the pan. Season with salt and pepper. Stir well to combine.
6. Simmer: Bring the curry to a simmer, then reduce the heat to low. Cover and let it simmer for 20-25 minutes, or until the eggplant is tender.
7. Adjust Seasoning: Taste and adjust the seasoning as needed. If you prefer more heat, you can add additional cayenne pepper.
8. Serve: Serve the Eggplant and Chickpea Curry over cooked rice or with naan.
9. Garnish and Enjoy: Garnish with fresh cilantro before serving. Enjoy your flavorful and hearty Eggplant and Chickpea Curry!

Spinach and Mushroom Quiche:

Ingredients:

For the Pie Crust:

- 1 1/4 cups all-purpose flour

- 1/2 cup unsalted butter, cold and diced

- 1/4 teaspoon salt

- 3-4 tablespoons ice water

For the Filling:

- 1 tablespoon olive oil
- 1 small onion, finely chopped
- 2 cups mushrooms, sliced

- 2 cups fresh spinach, chopped
- 1 clove garlic, minced
- 4 large eggs
- 1 cup milk
- Salt and pepper to taste
- 1/2 teaspoon dried thyme
- 1 1/2 cups shredded Swiss or Gruyere cheese

Instructions:

Prepare the Pie Crust:

1. Make Dough: In a food processor, combine flour, cold diced butter, and salt. Pulse until the mixture resembles coarse crumbs.
2. Add Water: Gradually add ice water, one tablespoon at a time, and pulse until the dough just comes together. Form the dough into a disc, wrap it in plastic wrap, and refrigerate for at least 30 minutes.
3. Roll Out Crust: Preheat the oven to 375°F (190°C). On a floured surface, roll out the chilled dough into a circle to fit your pie dish. Place the rolled-out dough in the pie dish and press it against the sides. Trim any excess dough.
4. Blind Bake (Optional): To prevent a soggy crust, you can blind bake the crust. Line the crust with parchment paper, fill with pie weights or dry beans, and bake for about 15 minutes. Remove the weights and parchment paper and bake for an additional 5 minutes until lightly golden.

Prepare the Filling:

1. Sauté Vegetables: In a skillet, heat olive oil over medium heat. Add chopped onion and sauté until softened. Add sliced mushrooms and cook until they release their moisture. Stir in chopped spinach and minced garlic, cooking until the spinach wilts. Allow the mixture to cool.
2. Whisk Eggs and Milk: In a bowl, whisk together eggs and milk. Season with salt, pepper, and dried thyme.
3. Assemble Quiche: Spread the sautéed vegetable mixture over the pre-baked crust. Sprinkle shredded cheese on top.
4. Pour Egg Mixture: Pour the egg and milk mixture over the vegetables and cheese.
5. Bake: Bake in the preheated oven for 35-40 minutes or until the center is set and the top is golden brown.
6. Cool and Serve: Allow the quiche to cool for a few minutes before slicing. Serve warm and enjoy your delicious Spinach and Mushroom Quiche!

Baked Salmon with Lemon and Dill:

Ingredients:

- 4 salmon filets (about 6 oz each) skin-on or skinless
- Salt and pepper to taste
- 2 tablespoons olive oil
- 2 tablespoons fresh dill, chopped
- 1 lemon, thinly sliced
- 2 cloves garlic, minced
- 1 tablespoon Dijon mustard
- 1 tablespoon honey or maple syrup (optional, for sweetness)

Instructions:

1. Preheat Oven: Preheat your oven to 400°F (200°C).
2. Prepare Salmon: Pat the salmon fillets dry with a paper towel. Season both sides with salt and pepper.
3. Mix Marinade: In a small bowl, whisk together olive oil, chopped dill, minced garlic, Dijon mustard, and honey or maple syrup (if using). This creates a flavorful marinade.
4. Marinate Salmon: Place the salmon fillets in a baking dish. Pour the marinade over the salmon, ensuring they are evenly coated. If you have skin-on salmon, make sure to get some of the marinade on the flesh as well.
5. Top with Lemon Slices: Lay lemon slices over the top of each salmon fillet. This adds brightness and flavor during baking.
6. Bake: Bake in the preheated oven for 12-15 minutes, or until the salmon is cooked through and flakes easily with a fork. The exact time may vary depending on the thickness of your salmon fillets.
7. Broil (Optional): For a golden top, you can broil the salmon for an additional 2-3 minutes after baking. Keep a close eye to avoid burning.

8. Serve: Once baked, carefully transfer the salmon fillets to serving plates. Spoon any remaining pan juices over the top.

9. Garnish (Optional): Garnish with additional fresh dill and lemon wedges.

10. Enjoy: Your Baked Salmon with Lemon and Dill is ready to be enjoyed. Serve it with your favorite sides for a delicious and healthy meal.

Quinoa and Vegetable Stir-Fry:

Ingredients:

- 1 cup quinoa, rinsed
- 2 cups water or vegetable broth
- 2 tablespoons soy sauce
- 1 tablespoon sesame oil
- 1 tablespoon olive oil
- 3 cloves garlic, minced
- 1 tablespoon fresh ginger, grated
- 1 medium carrot, julienned
- 1 bell pepper, thinly sliced (any color)
- 1 zucchini, thinly sliced
- 1 cup broccoli florets
- 1 cup snap peas, ends trimmed
- 2 green onions, chopped
- 1 tablespoon rice vinegar
- Salt and pepper to taste
- Sesame seeds for garnish (optional)

Instructions:

1. Prepare Quinoa: In a medium saucepan, combine quinoa and water or vegetable broth. Bring to a boil, then reduce heat to low, cover, and simmer for 15-20 minutes or until quinoa is cooked and water is absorbed.

2. Make Sauce: In a small bowl, whisk together soy sauce, sesame oil, and rice vinegar. Set aside.

3. Sauté Aromatics: In a large wok or skillet, heat olive oil over medium-high heat. Add minced garlic and grated ginger. Sauté for about 30 seconds until fragrant.

4. Add Vegetables: Add julienned carrot, sliced bell pepper, zucchini, broccoli florets, and snap peas to the wok. Stir-fry for 5-7 minutes or until the vegetables are crisp-tender.

5. Combine Quinoa and Sauce: Add cooked quinoa to the wok. Pour the prepared sauce over the quinoa and vegetables.

6. Toss and Season: Toss everything together to coat the quinoa and vegetables evenly with the sauce. Season with salt and pepper to taste.

7. Add Green Onions: Stir in chopped green onions and cook for an additional 1-2 minutes.

8. Garnish (Optional): If desired, garnish with sesame seeds for added texture and flavor.

9. Serve: Portion the Quinoa and Vegetable Stir-Fry into bowls or plates.

10. Enjoy: Your nutritious and delicious Quinoa and Vegetable Stir-Fry is ready to be enjoyed as a satisfying and flavorful meal.

Grilled Chicken and Asparagus:

Ingredients:

- 4 boneless, skinless chicken breasts
- 1 bunch fresh asparagus, woody ends trimmed
- 3 tablespoons olive oil
- 2 cloves garlic, minced
- 1 teaspoon lemon zest
- 2 tablespoons lemon juice
- 1 teaspoon dried oregano
- Salt and pepper to taste

- Fresh parsley for garnish (optional)

Instructions:

1. Preheat Grill: Preheat your grill to medium-high heat.
2. Prepare Chicken: Pat the chicken breasts dry with a paper towel. Season with salt and pepper.
3. Marinate Chicken: In a bowl, whisk together 2 tablespoons of olive oil, minced garlic, lemon zest, lemon juice, and dried oregano. Place the chicken breasts in the marinade, ensuring they are well coated. Let them marinate for at least 15-30 minutes.
4. Grill Chicken: Grill the marinated chicken breasts for 6-8 minutes per side, or until they reach an internal temperature of 165°F (74°C) and have beautiful grill marks. Cooking times may vary depending on the thickness of the chicken.
5. Prepare Asparagus: Toss the trimmed asparagus with the remaining 1 tablespoon of olive oil, salt, and pepper.
6. Grill Asparagus: Place the asparagus on the grill alongside the chicken during the last 5 minutes of cooking. Grill until the asparagus is tender-crisp and slightly charred.
7. Check Chicken Temperature: Ensure the chicken is fully cooked by checking the internal temperature with a meat thermometer.
8. Rest Chicken: Remove the chicken from the grill and let it rest for a few minutes. This allows the juices to redistribute, keeping the chicken moist.
9. Serve: Arrange the grilled chicken on a plate, and add the grilled asparagus on the side.
10. Garnish (Optional): Garnish with fresh parsley and serve your Grilled Chicken and Asparagus hot.

Mushroom and Spinach Stuffed Chicken Breast:

Ingredients:

- 4 boneless, skinless chicken breasts

- Salt and pepper to taste
- 1 tablespoon olive oil
- 8 oz mushrooms, finely chopped
- 2 cups fresh spinach, chopped
- 3 cloves garlic, minced
- 1/2 cup shredded mozzarella cheese
- 1/4 cup grated Parmesan cheese
- 1 teaspoon dried thyme
- 1 teaspoon dried rosemary
- 1/2 cup chicken broth
- Toothpicks or kitchen twine (optional)

Instructions:

1. Preheat Oven: Preheat your oven to 375°F (190°C).
2. Prepare Chicken: Lay the chicken breasts flat on a cutting board. Season both sides with salt and pepper.
3. Make Mushroom and Spinach Filling: In a skillet, heat olive oil over medium heat. Add chopped mushrooms and cook until they release their moisture and become golden brown. Add minced garlic and chopped spinach, cooking until the spinach wilts. Remove from heat.
4. Add Cheeses and Herbs: Stir in mozzarella and Parmesan cheeses, dried thyme, and dried rosemary into the mushroom and spinach mixture. Mix well until the cheese is melted.
5. Create Pocket in Chicken: Slice a pocket into each chicken breast. Be careful not to cut all the way through. You want to create a pocket for the stuffing.
6. Stuff Chicken: Stuff each chicken breast with a generous portion of the mushroom and spinach mixture.
7. Secure with Toothpicks or Twine (Optional): If needed, secure the pockets with toothpicks or tie with kitchen twine to keep the filling in place during cooking.

8. Season Outside of Chicken: Season the outside of each stuffed chicken breast with a bit more salt and pepper.

9. Sear Chicken: In an oven-safe skillet, sear the stuffed chicken breasts over medium-high heat for 2-3 minutes per side until they develop a golden brown crust.

10. Add Chicken Broth: Pour chicken broth into the skillet to keep the chicken moist during baking.

11. Bake: Transfer the skillet to the preheated oven and bake for 20-25 minutes or until the chicken reaches an internal temperature of 165°F (74°C).

12. Rest and Serve: Allow the stuffed chicken breasts to rest for a few minutes before serving. This helps retain their juices.

13. Serve: Slice the stuffed chicken breasts and serve with your favorite side dishes.

Veggie and Lentil Curry:

Ingredients:

- 1 cup dry lentils (red or green), rinsed and drained
- 1 tablespoon vegetable oil
- 1 large onion, finely chopped
- 3 cloves garlic, minced
- 1 tablespoon fresh ginger, grated
- 2 tablespoons curry powder
- 1 teaspoon ground cumin
- 1 teaspoon ground coriander
- 1/2 teaspoon turmeric
- 1/2 teaspoon cayenne pepper (adjust to taste)
- 1 can (14 oz) diced tomatoes
- 1 can (14 oz) coconut milk
- 3 cups mixed vegetables (e.g., carrots, bell peppers, peas, spinach)
- Salt and pepper to taste

- Fresh cilantro for garnish
- Cooked rice or naan for serving

Instructions:

1. Cook Lentils: In a medium saucepan, combine lentils with 2 cups of water. Bring to a boil, then reduce heat to low, cover, and simmer for 15-20 minutes or until lentils are tender. Drain any excess water.
2. Sauté Aromatics: In a large pot or deep skillet, heat vegetable oil over medium heat. Add chopped onion and sauté until softened. Add minced garlic and grated ginger, sauté for about 1-2 minutes until fragrant.
3. Add Spices: Stir in curry powder, ground cumin, ground coriander, turmeric, and cayenne pepper. Cook for 1-2 minutes to toast the spices.
4. Combine Tomatoes and Coconut Milk: Add diced tomatoes (with their juice) and coconut milk to the pot. Stir well to combine.
5. Add Lentils and Vegetables: Add the cooked lentils and mixed vegetables to the pot. If using frozen peas or spinach, add them in the last few minutes of cooking.
6. Simmer: Bring the curry to a simmer. Cover and let it simmer for 15-20 minutes to allow the flavors to meld and the vegetables to cook.
7. Season: Season the curry with salt and pepper to taste. Adjust the seasoning as needed.
8. Garnish: Garnish with fresh cilantro before serving.
9. Serve: Serve the Veggie and Lentil Curry over cooked rice or with naan.
10. Enjoy: Your hearty and nutritious Veggie and Lentil Curry is ready to be enjoyed as a flavorful and satisfying meal.

Turkey and Sweet Potato Skillet:

Ingredients:

- 1 lb ground turkey
- 2 tablespoons olive oil
- 1 onion, diced

- 2 cloves garlic, minced
- 2 medium sweet potatoes, peeled and diced
- 1 teaspoon ground cumin
- 1 teaspoon smoked paprika
- 1/2 teaspoon ground cinnamon
- Salt and pepper to taste
- 1 can (14 oz) diced tomatoes
- 1 cup black beans, drained and rinsed
- 1 cup corn kernels (fresh or frozen)
- 1 cup spinach, chopped
- 1/4 cup fresh cilantro, chopped (optional, for garnish)
- Lime wedges for serving

Instructions:

1. Cook Turkey: In a large skillet, brown the ground turkey over medium-high heat until fully cooked. Break it apart with a spoon as it cooks. Once done, remove excess fat if needed.
2. Sauté Aromatics: Add olive oil to the skillet. Sauté diced onion and minced garlic until softened.
3. Add Sweet Potatoes and Spices: Add diced sweet potatoes to the skillet. Sprinkle ground cumin, smoked paprika, ground cinnamon, salt, and pepper over the ingredients. Stir to combine.
4. Cook Sweet Potatoes: Cover the skillet and let the sweet potatoes cook for 8-10 minutes or until they are fork-tender, stirring occasionally.
5. Combine Tomatoes and Beans: Pour in the diced tomatoes (with their juice), black beans, and corn kernels. Stir well to combine.
6. Add Spinach: Add chopped spinach to the skillet. Stir until the spinach wilts and combines with the other ingredients.
7. Adjust Seasoning: Taste the mixture and adjust the seasoning with salt and pepper as needed.

8. Garnish (Optional): If desired, garnish with fresh cilantro.

9. Serve: Serve the Turkey and Sweet Potato Skillet hot.

10. Enjoy: Squeeze lime wedges over individual servings for a burst of freshness. Enjoy this wholesome and flavorful Turkey and Sweet Potato Skillet.

Cauliflower and Chickpea Coconut Curry:

Ingredients:

- 1 tablespoon vegetable oil
- 1 onion, finely chopped
- 3 cloves garlic, minced
- 1 tablespoon fresh ginger, grated
- 1 cauliflower, cut into florets
- 1 can (15 oz) chickpeas, drained and rinsed
- 1 can (14 oz) diced tomatoes
- 1 can (14 oz) coconut milk
- 2 tablespoons curry powder
- 1 teaspoon ground turmeric
- 1 teaspoon ground cumin
- 1 teaspoon ground coriander
- 1/2 teaspoon red pepper flakes (adjust to taste)
- Salt and pepper to taste
- Fresh cilantro for garnish
- Cooked rice for serving

Instructions:

1. Sauté Aromatics: In a large pot or deep skillet, heat vegetable oil over medium heat. Add chopped onion and sauté until softened. Add minced garlic and grated ginger, sauté for about 1-2 minutes until fragrant.

2. Add Cauliflower and Chickpeas: Add cauliflower florets and drained chickpeas to the pot. Stir to combine with the aromatics.

3. Pour in Tomatoes and Coconut Milk: Add diced tomatoes (with their juice) and coconut milk to the pot. Stir well.

4. Add Spices: Sprinkle curry powder, ground turmeric, ground cumin, ground coriander, red pepper flakes, salt, and pepper over the mixture. Stir to evenly distribute the spices.

5. Simmer: Bring the curry to a simmer. Cover and let it simmer for 15-20 minutes or until the cauliflower is tender.

6. Adjust Seasoning: Taste the curry and adjust the seasoning if needed. If you prefer more heat, you can add additional red pepper flakes.

7. Garnish: Garnish with fresh cilantro just before serving.

8. Serve: Serve the Cauliflower and Chickpea Coconut Curry over cooked rice.

9. Enjoy: Your flavorful and creamy Cauliflower and Chickpea Coconut Curry is ready to be enjoyed as a delicious and satisfying meal.

Eggplant and Tomato Stew:

Ingredients:

- 1 large eggplant, diced
- 2 tablespoons olive oil
- 1 onion, finely chopped
- 3 cloves garlic, minced
- 1 can (14 oz) diced tomatoes
- 1 can (6 oz) tomato paste
- 1 cup vegetable broth
- 1 teaspoon dried oregano
- 1 teaspoon dried basil
- 1/2 teaspoon dried thyme
- Salt and pepper to taste
- 1/4 cup fresh parsley, chopped (for garnish)
- Grated Parmesan cheese (optional, for serving)

- Cooked rice or crusty bread for serving

Instructions:

1. Prepare Eggplant: Place diced eggplant in a colander, sprinkle with salt, and let it sit for about 20 minutes. This helps draw out excess moisture and bitterness. Rinse and pat dry with paper towels.
2. Sauté Aromatics: In a large pot or deep skillet, heat olive oil over medium heat. Add chopped onion and sauté until softened. Add minced garlic and sauté for about 1-2 minutes until fragrant.
3. Add Eggplant: Add the prepared eggplant to the pot. Sauté until it begins to brown.
4. Stir in Tomatoes and Tomato Paste: Pour in diced tomatoes (with their juice) and tomato paste. Stir well to combine.
5. Add Broth and Herbs: Pour vegetable broth into the pot. Add dried oregano, dried basil, dried thyme, salt, and pepper. Stir to incorporate.
6. Simmer: Bring the stew to a simmer. Cover and let it simmer for 20-25 minutes, or until the eggplant is tender and the flavors meld.
7. Adjust Seasoning: Taste and adjust the seasoning as needed. Add more salt and pepper if required.
8. Garnish: Garnish the Eggplant and Tomato Stew with fresh parsley just before serving.
9. Serve: Serve the stew over cooked rice or with crusty bread. Optionally, sprinkle with grated Parmesan cheese.
10. Enjoy: Your hearty and flavorful Eggplant and Tomato Stew is ready to be enjoyed as a comforting and satisfying meal.

Shrimp and Avocado Salad:

Ingredients:

For the Shrimp:

- 1 lb large shrimp, peeled and deveined

- 2 tablespoons olive oil
- 2 cloves garlic, minced
- 1 teaspoon paprika
- Salt and pepper to taste
- Fresh lemon wedges for serving

For the Salad:

- 4 cups mixed salad greens (e.g., spinach, arugula, or mixed greens)
- 2 ripe avocados, sliced
- 1 cup cherry tomatoes, halved
- 1 cucumber, sliced
- 1/4 red onion, thinly sliced

For the Dressing:

- 3 tablespoons olive oil
- 2 tablespoons fresh lemon juice
- 1 teaspoon Dijon mustard
- 1 clove garlic, minced
- Salt and pepper to taste

Instructions:

Prepare Shrimp:

1. Season Shrimp: In a bowl, toss the peeled and deveined shrimp with olive oil, minced garlic, paprika, salt, and pepper.
2. Sauté Shrimp: In a skillet over medium-high heat, cook the seasoned shrimp for 2-3 minutes per side or until they are pink and opaque. Remove from heat.
3. Serve: Squeeze fresh lemon juice over the cooked shrimp before serving.

Prepare Salad:

1. Assemble Greens: Arrange the mixed salad greens on a serving platter or individual plates.
2. Add Vegetables: Top the greens with sliced avocados, halved cherry tomatoes, cucumber slices, and thinly sliced red onion.

Prepare Dressing:

1. Whisk Dressing: In a small bowl, whisk together olive oil, fresh lemon juice, Dijon mustard, minced garlic, salt, and pepper.
2. Drizzle Dressing: Drizzle the dressing over the salad.

Assemble and Serve:

1. Add Shrimp: Place the cooked shrimp on top of the salad.
2. Garnish: Garnish the Shrimp and Avocado Salad with additional lemon wedges and fresh herbs if desired.
3. Serve: Serve the salad immediately, and enjoy the vibrant flavors of this refreshing and satisfying dish.

Spinach and Feta Stuffed Portobello Mushrooms:

Ingredients:

- 4 large Portobello mushrooms, stems removed and cleaned
- 2 tablespoons olive oil
- 2 cloves garlic, minced
- 4 cups fresh spinach, chopped
- 1/2 cup crumbled feta cheese
- 1/4 cup grated Parmesan cheese
- Salt and pepper to taste
- 1 teaspoon dried oregano
- 1 teaspoon dried thyme
- Balsamic glaze for drizzling (optional)
- Fresh parsley for garnish (optional)

Instructions:

1. Prepare Mushrooms: Preheat the oven to 375°F (190°C). Line a baking sheet with parchment paper. Clean the Portobello mushrooms, remove the stems, and place them on the baking sheet.

2. Sauté Spinach: In a large skillet, heat olive oil over medium heat. Add minced garlic and sauté until fragrant. Add chopped spinach and cook until wilted. Season with salt and pepper.

3. Combine Spinach and Cheese: In a bowl, mix the sautéed spinach with crumbled feta cheese, grated Parmesan, dried oregano, and dried thyme. Adjust seasoning to taste.

4. Stuff Mushrooms: Spoon the spinach and cheese mixture into the cavity of each Portobello mushroom, pressing down gently.

5. Bake: Bake in the preheated oven for 20-25 minutes or until the mushrooms are tender and the filling is heated through.

6. Optional Broil: If desired, you can broil the stuffed mushrooms for an additional 2-3 minutes to get a golden top.

7. Drizzle with Balsamic Glaze: Before serving, drizzle with balsamic glaze for added flavor (optional).

8. Garnish: Garnish with fresh parsley if desired.

9. Serve: Serve the Spinach and Feta Stuffed Portobello Mushrooms as a tasty appetizer or a light main dish.

Lemon Herb Baked Cod:

Ingredients:

- 4 cod fillets (about 6 oz each)
- 2 tablespoons olive oil
- 2 tablespoons fresh lemon juice
- 2 cloves garlic, minced
- 1 teaspoon fresh thyme, chopped
- 1 teaspoon fresh rosemary, chopped
- 1 teaspoon fresh parsley, chopped
- Zest of one lemon
- Salt and pepper to taste

- Lemon slices for garnish
- Fresh parsley for garnish

Instructions:

1. Preheat Oven: Preheat your oven to 400°F (200°C). Line a baking dish with parchment paper.
2. Prepare Cod Fillets: Pat the cod fillets dry with a paper towel. Place them in the prepared baking dish.
3. Make Herb Marinade: In a small bowl, whisk together olive oil, fresh lemon juice, minced garlic, chopped thyme, chopped rosemary, chopped parsley, lemon zest, salt, and pepper.
4. Marinate Cod: Pour the herb marinade over the cod fillets, ensuring they are well coated on both sides. Let them marinate for 15-20 minutes for the flavors to infuse.
5. Bake: Bake the cod fillets in the preheated oven for 12-15 minutes or until the fish is opaque and flakes easily with a fork.
6. Broil (Optional): If you desire a golden top, you can broil the cod for an additional 2-3 minutes, keeping a close eye to avoid burning.
7. Garnish and Serve: Garnish the Lemon Herb Baked Cod with lemon slices and fresh parsley.
8. Serve: Serve the baked cod fillets hot with your favorite side dishes.

Chickpea and Vegetable Tagine

Ingredients:

- 1 can (15 oz) chickpeas, drained and rinsed
- 2 tablespoons olive oil
- 1 onion, finely chopped
- 2 cloves garlic, minced
- 1 teaspoon ground cumin
- 1 teaspoon ground coriander
- 1 teaspoon ground cinnamon
- 1/2 teaspoon ground turmeric

- 1/2 teaspoon paprika
- 1/4 teaspoon cayenne pepper (adjust to taste)
- 1 eggplant, diced
- 2 zucchinis, diced
- 2 carrots, peeled and sliced
- 1 red bell pepper, diced
- 1 can (14 oz) diced tomatoes
- 1 cup vegetable broth
- 1/2 cup dried apricots, chopped
- Salt and pepper to taste
- Fresh cilantro or parsley for garnish
- Cooked couscous or rice for serving

Instructions:

1. Sauté Aromatics: In a large, heavy-bottomed pot or tagine, heat olive oil over medium heat. Add chopped onion and sauté until softened. Add minced garlic and sauté for an additional 1-2 minutes until fragrant.
2. Add Spices: Add ground cumin, ground coriander, ground cinnamon, ground turmeric, paprika, and cayenne pepper to the pot. Stir well to coat the onions and garlic in the spices.
3. Add Vegetables: Add diced eggplant, zucchinis, carrots, and red bell pepper to the pot. Cook for 5-7 minutes until the vegetables begin to soften.
4. Incorporate Chickpeas: Stir in the drained and rinsed chickpeas, mixing them with the vegetables.
5. Pour in Tomatoes and Broth: Add diced tomatoes (with their juice) and vegetable broth to the pot. Stir to combine.
6. Simmer: Bring the mixture to a simmer. Cover and let it simmer for 15-20 minutes, allowing the flavors to meld and the vegetables to become tender.
7. Add Dried Apricots: Add chopped dried apricots to the tagine, stirring them in. This adds sweetness and a delightful flavor.
8. Season: Season the tagine with salt and pepper to taste. Adjust the seasoning as needed.
9. Garnish and Serve: Garnish the Chickpea and Vegetable Tagine with fresh cilantro or parsley just before serving. Serve the tagine over cooked couscous or rice.
10. Enjoy: Your delicious and aromatic Chickpea and Vegetable Tagine is ready to be enjoyed as a hearty and flavorful meal.

CHAPTER 6: SNACKS AND APPETIZERS

Almonds and Berries:

Ingredients:

- 1 cup mixed berries (strawberries, blueberries, raspberries)
- 1/2 cup almonds, sliced or whole
- 1 tablespoon honey or maple syrup (optional)
- Greek yogurt or your favorite yogurt (optional)

Instructions:

1. Prepare Berries: Wash and prepare the berries as needed. If using strawberries, hull and slice them.
2. Toast Almonds: In a dry skillet over medium heat, toast the almonds until they become golden and fragrant. Stir frequently to prevent burning. This usually takes about 3-5 minutes.
3. Combine Berries and Almonds: In a bowl, combine the mixed berries with the toasted almonds.
4. Optional Sweetener: If you desire added sweetness, drizzle honey or maple syrup over the berries and almonds. Toss gently to coat.
5. Serve with Yogurt (Optional): If you enjoy yogurt, serve the almond and berry mixture over a bed of Greek yogurt or your favorite yogurt.
6. Enjoy: This Almonds and Berries recipe is a simple and delicious way to enjoy the natural sweetness of berries combined with the crunch of toasted almonds. It can be served as a snack, breakfast, or a healthy dessert.

Greek Yogurt with Honey:

Ingredients:

- 1 cup Greek yogurt
- 2 tablespoons honey (adjust to taste)
- Fresh berries or sliced fruit (optional)

- Chopped nuts (e.g., almonds, walnuts) for garnish (optional)
- Mint leaves for garnish (optional)

Instructions:

1. Spoon Greek Yogurt: Measure out 1 cup of Greek yogurt and spoon it into a serving bowl.

2. Drizzle Honey: Drizzle 2 tablespoons of honey over the Greek yogurt. Adjust the amount based on your desired level of sweetness.

3. Swirl or Mix: Use a spoon to gently swirl the honey into the Greek yogurt, ensuring it's evenly distributed. You can also mix it if you prefer a more uniform flavor.

4. Add Fresh Fruit (Optional): Enhance your Greek Yogurt with fresh berries or sliced fruit. Berries like strawberries, blueberries, or raspberries work well.

5. Garnish with Nuts (Optional): For added texture and flavor, sprinkle chopped nuts, such as almonds or walnuts, over the yogurt.

6. Garnish with Mint (Optional): Add a touch of freshness by garnishing with mint leaves.

7. Serve: Enjoy your delicious Greek Yogurt with Honey immediately as a nutritious and satisfying snack or breakfast.

Carrot Sticks with Hummus:

Ingredients:

- Fresh carrots, peeled and cut into sticks
- Hummus (store-bought or homemade)
- Optional: Olive oil, paprika, sesame seeds, or fresh herbs for garnish

Instructions:

1. Prepare Carrot Sticks: Wash, peel, and cut fresh carrots into sticks. The size can vary based on your preference.

2. Serve with Hummus: Arrange the carrot sticks on a serving plate or platter. Place a bowl of hummus in the center or on the side for dipping.

3. Garnish (Optional): Drizzle a bit of olive oil over the hummus. Sprinkle it with paprika, sesame seeds, or fresh herbs like parsley for added flavor and visual appeal.

4. Serve and Enjoy: Serve the carrot sticks with hummus immediately. Enjoy the crispness of the carrots combined with the creamy and flavorful hummus.

Apple Slices with Almond Butter:

Ingredients:

- Fresh apples (your favorite variety)
- Almond butter (store-bought or homemade)
- Optional toppings: Chia seeds, sliced almonds, or a drizzle of honey

Instructions:

1. Prepare Apples: Wash and core the apples. Slice them into thin wedges or rounds. You can leave the peel on for added nutrition and texture.

2. Serve with Almond Butter: Place a dollop of almond butter in a small bowl or on a serving plate. You can use store-bought almond butter or make your own by blending almonds until smooth.

3. Dip and Spread: Dip the apple slices into the almond butter, ensuring each slice is coated with creamy goodness. Alternatively, you can spread almond butter directly onto the apple slices.

4. Optional Toppings: For added crunch and flavor, sprinkle chia seeds, sliced almonds, or drizzle a bit of honey over the apple slices and almond butter.

5. Serve and Enjoy: Arrange the apple slices on a platter or enjoy them right from the bowl. This simple and nutritious snack is ready to be savored.

Dark Chocolate Covered Strawberries:

Ingredients:

- Fresh strawberries, washed and dried
- Dark chocolate chips or chopped dark chocolate (70% cocoa or higher)

- White chocolate (optional, for drizzling)
- Toppings (optional): Chopped nuts, shredded coconut, or sprinkles

Instructions:

1. Prepare Strawberries: Wash and thoroughly dry the strawberries. Make sure they are completely dry to help the chocolate adhere better.

2. Melt Dark Chocolate: Place the dark chocolate chips or chopped dark chocolate in a heatproof bowl. Microwave in 20-second intervals, stirring between each, until the chocolate is fully melted. Alternatively, you can melt the chocolate using a double boiler.

3. Dip Strawberries: Hold each strawberry by the stem and dip it into the melted dark chocolate, making sure to coat it evenly. Allow excess chocolate to drip off.

4. Place on Parchment Paper: Place the chocolate-covered strawberries on a parchment paper-lined tray or plate. This will prevent them from sticking and make cleanup easier.

5. Optional White Chocolate Drizzle: If desired, melt white chocolate using the same method as the dark chocolate. Drizzle it over the dipped strawberries for an additional decorative touch.

6. Add Toppings (Optional): While the chocolate is still wet, sprinkle chopped nuts, shredded coconut, or colorful sprinkles over the strawberries.

7. Chill: Place the tray of chocolate-covered strawberries in the refrigerator to allow the chocolate to set. This usually takes about 30 minutes to an hour.

8. Serve and Enjoy: Once the chocolate is set, remove the strawberries from the refrigerator. Arrange them on a serving platter, and they are ready to be enjoyed.

Cherry Tomatoes and Mozzarella Balls:

Ingredients:

- Cherry tomatoes, washed
- Fresh mozzarella balls (bocconcini), drained
- Fresh basil leaves

- Extra-virgin olive oil
- Balsamic glaze (optional)
- Salt and pepper to taste

Instructions:

1. Prepare Ingredients: Wash the cherry tomatoes and drain the fresh mozzarella balls. Set aside fresh basil leaves.
2. Assemble Salad: On a serving platter or in a bowl, arrange the cherry tomatoes and mozzarella balls. You can alternate them for a visually appealing presentation.
3. Add Basil Leaves: Tuck fresh basil leaves among the cherry tomatoes and mozzarella balls. Tear the leaves if you prefer a more rustic look.
4. Drizzle with Olive Oil: Drizzle extra-virgin olive oil over the salad. Use a good quality olive oil for enhanced flavor.
5. Season with Salt and Pepper: Sprinkle salt and pepper over the salad to taste. Remember that the mozzarella may already contain some salt, so adjust accordingly.
6. Optional Balsamic Glaze: For a sweet and tangy touch, you can drizzle balsamic glaze over the salad. This step is optional but adds a delightful flavor.
7. Toss Gently (Optional): If you prefer, gently toss the ingredients to coat them in the olive oil and seasoning. Be careful not to crush the mozzarella balls.
8. Serve: Your Cherry Tomatoes and Mozzarella Balls Salad is ready to be served. It's a refreshing and flavorful dish, perfect as a side or a light appetizer.

Celery with Peanut Butter:

Ingredients:

- Fresh celery stalks, washed and trimmed
- Peanut butter (smooth or crunchy)

Instructions:

1. Prepare Celery: Wash the celery stalks thoroughly and trim off the ends. Optionally, cut the stalks into manageable lengths.

2. Spread Peanut Butter: Using a butter knife or a spoon, spread peanut butter along the concave side of each celery stalk.

3. Optional Variations: You can customize this snack by adding toppings such as raisins (for "Ants on a Log"), sliced bananas, or a sprinkle of cinnamon for extra flavor.

4. Serve: Arrange the celery sticks on a plate or tray and serve immediately.

Edamame:

Ingredients:

- 1 pound (about 2 cups) fresh or frozen edamame in the pod
- 1-2 teaspoons sea salt (for boiling)

Instructions:

1. Prepare Edamame:
   - If using frozen edamame, thaw them if necessary.
   - Rinse fresh or thawed edamame under cold water.

2. Boil Water:
   - Fill a large pot with water and bring it to a boil.

3. Boil Edamame:
   - Add 1-2 teaspoons of sea salt to the boiling water.
   - Add the edamame to the boiling water.
   - Cook for 4-5 minutes for fresh edamame or 2-3 minutes for frozen edamame. They should be tender but still have a slight crunch.

4. Drain and Cool:
   - Drain the edamame in a colander and rinse them under cold water. This stops the cooking process and helps retain their vibrant green color.

5. Serve:
   - Serve the edamame in a bowl, and they are ready to be enjoyed.

Optional Seasonings:

- Salted Edamame: Sprinkle with additional sea salt to taste.

- Spicy Edamame: Toss with a mixture of soy sauce, sesame oil, and a pinch of red pepper flakes.
- Garlic Edamame: Sauté cooked edamame in a pan with minced garlic and a drizzle of olive oil.
- Sesame Edamame: Drizzle with sesame oil and sprinkle sesame seeds.

Mixed Nuts:

Ingredients:

- 2 cups mixed nuts (almonds, walnuts, cashews, pecans, etc.)
- 1 tablespoon olive oil or melted butter
- 1 teaspoon salt (adjust to taste)
- 1/2 teaspoon garlic powder (optional)
- 1/2 teaspoon onion powder (optional)
- 1/2 teaspoon paprika (optional)
- 1/4 teaspoon cayenne pepper (optional for heat)
- 1 tablespoon honey (optional, for a touch of sweetness)

Instructions:

1. Preheat Oven:
   - Preheat your oven to 350°F (175°C).
2. Mix Nuts:
   - In a bowl, combine the mixed nuts with olive oil or melted butter, ensuring they are evenly coated.
3. Season:
   - Add salt and any optional seasonings such as garlic powder, onion powder, paprika, cayenne pepper, or honey. Toss the nuts to coat them evenly with the seasonings.
4. Spread on Baking Sheet:
   - Spread the seasoned nuts in a single layer on a baking sheet lined with parchment paper.

5. Roast:
   o Roast the mixed nuts in the preheated oven for 10-15 minutes, or until they become golden brown and fragrant. Stir the nuts halfway through the roasting time for even browning.
6. Cool:
   o Allow the roasted mixed nuts to cool on the baking sheet for a few minutes. They will continue to crisp up as they cool.
7. Serve:
   o Once cooled, transfer the mixed nuts to a serving bowl.

Avocado and Whole Grain Crackers:

Ingredients:

- 2 ripe avocados
- Whole grain crackers
- Lemon or lime juice (optional, to prevent avocado from browning)
- Salt and pepper to taste
- Red pepper flakes (optional, for added spice)
- Fresh cilantro or parsley for garnish (optional)

Instructions:

1. Prepare Avocado:
   o Cut the avocados in half, remove the pits, and scoop the flesh into a bowl.
2. Mash Avocado:
   o Mash the avocado with a fork until it reaches your desired level of smoothness.
3. Season:
   o Add salt and pepper to taste. Optionally, squeeze a bit of lemon or lime juice over the mashed avocado to prevent browning and add a citrusy flavor.
4. Assemble:

- Spread the mashed avocado onto whole grain crackers. Use as much or as little avocado as you prefer.

5. Optional Garnishes:
   - Sprinkle red pepper flakes for a touch of spice.
   - Garnish with fresh cilantro or parsley for added freshness.

6. Serve:
   - Arrange the avocado-topped crackers on a plate and serve immediately.

Berries and Cottage Cheese:

Ingredients:

- 1 cup cottage cheese
- 1 cup mixed berries (strawberries, blueberries, raspberries, blackberries)
- 1 tablespoon honey or maple syrup (optional)
- 1/4 cup granola (optional, for crunch)
- Fresh mint leaves for garnish (optional)

Instructions:

1. Prepare Berries:
   - Wash and prepare the berries as needed. If using strawberries, hull and slice them.
2. Assemble Cottage Cheese:
   - Spoon the cottage cheese into a serving bowl.
3. Add Berries:
   - Top the cottage cheese with the mixed berries.
4. Drizzle Sweetener (Optional):
   - If desired, drizzle honey or maple syrup over the berries and cottage cheese for added sweetness.
5. Sprinkle Granola (Optional):
   - For extra crunch, sprinkle granola over the top of the berries and cottage cheese.

6. Garnish with Mint (Optional):

   o Garnish the bowl with fresh mint leaves for a burst of freshness.

7. Serve Immediately:

   o Serve the Berries and Cottage Cheese bowl immediately, and enjoy!

Popcorn with Turmeric:

Ingredients:

- 1/2 cup popcorn kernels
- 2 tablespoons coconut oil or olive oil
- 1 teaspoon ground turmeric
- 1/2 teaspoon paprika (optional, for added flavor)
- Salt to taste

Instructions:

1. Pop the Popcorn:

   o Pop the popcorn kernels using your preferred method (air popper, stovetop, or microwave).

2. Prepare Turmeric Mixture:

   o In a small saucepan, melt the coconut oil or heat the olive oil over low heat. Add ground turmeric and paprika (if using). Stir well to combine.

3. Drizzle over Popcorn:

   o Drizzle the turmeric mixture over the popped popcorn. Toss the popcorn gently to ensure even coating.

4. Season with Salt:

   o Sprinkle salt over the turmeric-coated popcorn to taste. Toss again to distribute the seasoning.

5. Serve:

   o Transfer the Turmeric Popcorn to a large bowl and serve immediately.

Roasted Chickpeas:

Ingredients:

- 2 cans (15 oz each) chickpeas, drained and rinsed
- 2 tablespoons olive oil
- 1 teaspoon ground cumin
- 1 teaspoon smoked paprika
- 1/2 teaspoon garlic powder
- 1/2 teaspoon onion powder
- 1/4 teaspoon cayenne pepper (adjust to taste)
- Salt and pepper to taste

Instructions:

1. Preheat your oven to 400°F (200°C) and line a baking sheet with parchment paper.
2. Pat the chickpeas dry with a clean kitchen towel or paper towels. Remove any loose skins for a crispier result.
3. In a bowl, combine the chickpeas, olive oil, cumin, smoked paprika, garlic powder, onion powder, cayenne pepper, salt, and pepper. Toss until the chickpeas are evenly coated.
4. Spread the seasoned chickpeas in a single layer on the prepared baking sheet.
5. Roast in the preheated oven for 25-30 minutes, shaking the pan halfway through to ensure even roasting. The chickpeas are done when they are golden brown and crispy.
6. Remove from the oven and let them cool for a few minutes. They will continue to crisp up as they cool.
7. Once cooled, store the roasted chickpeas in an airtight container. Enjoy them as a snack, salad topper, or crunchy addition to your favorite dishes.

APPETIZERS:

Stuffed Bell Peppers with Quinoa:

Ingredients:

- 4 large bell peppers, any color
- 1 cup quinoa, rinsed and cooked according to package instructions
- 1 tablespoon olive oil
- 1 onion, finely chopped
- 2 cloves garlic, minced
- 1 zucchini, diced
- 1 cup cherry tomatoes, halved
- 1 cup black beans, drained and rinsed
- 1 teaspoon ground cumin
- 1 teaspoon smoked paprika
- Salt and pepper to taste
- 1 cup shredded cheese (cheddar, mozzarella, or your choice)
- Fresh parsley or cilantro for garnish (optional)

Instructions:

1. Preheat your oven to 375°F (190°C).
2. Cut the tops off the bell peppers and remove the seeds and membranes. Lightly brush the outside of the peppers with olive oil and place them in a baking dish.
3. In a large skillet, heat 1 tablespoon of olive oil over medium heat. Add the chopped onion and garlic, sautéing until softened.
4. Add diced zucchini to the skillet and cook until it begins to soften. Then, stir in the halved cherry tomatoes and black beans.
5. Incorporate the cooked quinoa into the vegetable mixture. Season with ground cumin, smoked paprika, salt, and pepper. Mix well.
6. Spoon the quinoa and vegetable mixture into each bell pepper, pressing down gently.

7. Top each stuffed pepper with shredded cheese.

8. Bake in the preheated oven for 25-30 minutes or until the peppers are tender, and the cheese is melted and bubbly.

9. Remove from the oven and let them cool for a few minutes before serving.

10. Garnish with fresh parsley or cilantro if desired. Serve the stuffed bell peppers with a side of your favorite sauce or salsa.

Caprese Skewers:

Ingredients:

- Cherry tomatoes
- Fresh mozzarella balls (bocconcini)
- Fresh basil leaves
- Balsamic glaze (store-bought or homemade)
- Extra virgin olive oil
- Salt and pepper to taste
- Wooden skewers

Instructions:

1. Assemble the ingredients for easy access.

2. Rinse the cherry tomatoes and basil leaves. Drain the fresh mozzarella balls if they are in liquid.

3. Take a wooden skewer and thread a cherry tomato onto it, followed by a folded basil leaf, and then a mozzarella ball.

4. Repeat the process for the desired number of skewers.

5. Arrange the assembled Caprese skewers on a serving platter.

6. Drizzle extra virgin olive oil over the skewers. Sprinkle with salt and pepper to taste.

7. Just before serving, generously drizzle balsamic glaze over the skewers. If you don't have balsamic glaze, you can reduce balsamic vinegar in a saucepan until it thickens.

8. Serve immediately as an appetizer or a refreshing snack.

Smoked Salmon Cucumber Bites:

Ingredients:

- English cucumbers, sliced into rounds
- Smoked salmon slices
- Cream cheese, softened
- Fresh dill, chopped
- Lemon zest
- Salt and pepper to taste
- Optional: Capers for garnish

Instructions:

1. Slice the English cucumbers into rounds, approximately 1/2 inch thick.
2. In a small bowl, mix the softened cream cheese with chopped fresh dill, lemon zest, salt, and pepper. Adjust the seasonings to your taste.
3. Spread a small amount of the cream cheese mixture onto each cucumber round.
4. Place a slice of smoked salmon on top of the cream cheese-covered cucumber.
5. Garnish each bite with additional fresh dill and, if desired, capers.
6. Arrange the smoked salmon cucumber bites on a serving platter.
7. Serve chilled and enjoy these elegant and refreshing appetizers.

Eggplant and Tomato Bruschetta:

Ingredients:

- 1 medium-sized eggplant, diced
- 1 pint cherry tomatoes, halved
- 2 cloves garlic, minced
- 1/4 cup fresh basil, chopped
- 1/4 cup extra virgin olive oil
- 1 tablespoon balsamic vinegar

- Salt and pepper to taste
- Baguette or Italian bread, sliced

Instructions:

1. Preheat the oven to 400°F (200°C).
2. Place the diced eggplant on a baking sheet. Drizzle with olive oil, and season with salt and pepper. Toss to coat evenly.
3. Roast the eggplant in the preheated oven for about 20-25 minutes or until golden and tender, stirring halfway through.
4. While the eggplant is roasting, mix together the halved cherry tomatoes, minced garlic, chopped basil, balsamic vinegar, and a bit more olive oil in a bowl. Season with salt and pepper to taste.
5. Once the eggplant is done, allow it to cool for a few minutes before combining it with the tomato mixture.
6. Toast the sliced baguette or Italian bread in the oven or on a grill until slightly crisp.
7. Spoon the eggplant and tomato mixture generously onto each slice of toasted bread.
8. Optionally, garnish with additional fresh basil.
9. Serve the eggplant and tomato bruschetta as a delightful appetizer or snack.

Guacamole with Veggie Sticks:

Ingredients:

- 3 ripe avocados
- 1 small red onion, finely diced
- 1-2 tomatoes, diced
- 1 jalapeño, seeded and finely minced
- 1-2 cloves garlic, minced
- Juice of 1-2 limes
- 1/4 cup fresh cilantro, chopped

- Salt and pepper to taste
- Assorted veggie sticks (carrots, cucumber, bell peppers) for dipping

Instructions:

1. Cut the avocados in half, remove the pits, and scoop the flesh into a bowl.
2. Mash the avocados with a fork or potato masher until you achieve your desired guacamole consistency (smooth or slightly chunky).
3. Add the finely diced red onion, diced tomatoes, minced jalapeño, minced garlic, and chopped cilantro to the mashed avocados.
4. Squeeze the juice of one lime into the mixture. Adjust the lime juice, salt, and pepper to taste.
5. Mix all the ingredients until well combined.
6. Taste and add more lime, salt, or pepper if needed.
7. Cover the guacamole with plastic wrap, pressing it directly onto the surface to minimize browning. Refrigerate until ready to serve.
8. Wash and cut assorted veggies into sticks.
9. Just before serving, give the guacamole a quick stir and adjust the seasoning if necessary.
10. Arrange the guacamole in a serving bowl and surround it with the veggie sticks for a colorful and healthy snack.

Shrimp Cocktail:

Ingredients:

- 1 pound large shrimp, peeled and deveined
- 1 lemon, sliced
- Cocktail sauce (store-bought or homemade)
- Fresh parsley, chopped, for garnish

For the Poaching Liquid:

- 4 cups water
- 1 bay leaf

- 1 teaspoon whole black peppercorns
- 1 teaspoon salt
- Ice water bath (for cooling shrimp)

For Homemade Cocktail Sauce:

- 1/2 cup ketchup
- 2 tablespoons horseradish (adjust to taste)
- 1 tablespoon lemon juice
- 1 teaspoon Worcestershire sauce
- Hot sauce to taste (optional)
- Salt and pepper to taste

Instructions:

1. In a large saucepan, combine water, bay leaf, peppercorns, and salt for the poaching liquid. Bring it to a simmer.
2. Add the peeled and deveined shrimp to the simmering liquid and cook for 3-4 minutes or until the shrimp turn pink and opaque.
3. Immediately transfer the cooked shrimp to an ice water bath to cool rapidly. Once cooled, drain and pat them dry with a paper towel.
4. In a bowl, mix together ketchup, horseradish, lemon juice, Worcestershire sauce, hot sauce (if using), salt, and pepper to prepare the cocktail sauce. Adjust the horseradish and hot sauce to your preferred level of spiciness.
5. Chill the cocktail sauce in the refrigerator until ready to serve.
6. Arrange the chilled shrimp on a serving platter with lemon slices for garnish.
7. Place the cocktail sauce in a bowl in the center of the platter or in individual serving cups.
8. Sprinkle chopped fresh parsley over the shrimp for a vibrant finish.
9. Serve the shrimp cocktail immediately as an appetizer or part of a seafood spread.

Hummus and Whole Wheat Pita Bread:

Ingredients:

For Hummus:

- 1 can (15 oz) chickpeas, drained and rinsed
- 1/4 cup tahini
- 2 cloves garlic, minced
- 2 tablespoons lemon juice
- 3 tablespoons extra virgin olive oil
- 1/2 teaspoon ground cumin
- Salt to taste
- Water (as needed for desired consistency)

For Whole Wheat Pita Bread:

- 2 cups whole wheat flour
- 1 teaspoon active dry yeast
- 1 teaspoon sugar
- 3/4 cup warm water
- 1 tablespoon olive oil
- 1/2 teaspoon salt

Instructions:

For Hummus:

1. In a food processor, combine chickpeas, tahini, minced garlic, lemon juice, olive oil, ground cumin, and a pinch of salt.
2. Blend until smooth, adding water gradually until you reach your desired consistency.
3. Taste and adjust salt and lemon juice as needed.
4. Transfer the hummus to a serving bowl, drizzle with a bit of olive oil, and garnish with a sprinkle of cumin or paprika if desired.

For Whole Wheat Pita Bread:

1. In a small bowl, combine warm water, sugar, and yeast. Let it sit for about 5 minutes until it becomes frothy.

2. In a large mixing bowl, combine whole wheat flour and salt. Make a well in the center and add the yeast mixture and olive oil.

3. Mix the ingredients until a dough forms, then knead on a floured surface for about 5-7 minutes, or until the dough becomes smooth and elastic.

4. Place the dough in a lightly oiled bowl, cover with a damp cloth, and let it rise in a warm place for 1-2 hours, or until it doubles in size.

5. Preheat your oven to 475°F (245°C).

6. Punch down the risen dough and divide it into small balls. Roll each ball into a thin round pita shape.

7. Place the rolled-out pitas on a baking sheet and bake for 5-7 minutes, or until they puff up and the edges turn golden.

8. Remove from the oven and let them cool slightly.

Serve:

1. Cut the whole wheat pita into wedges.

2. Arrange the pita wedges around a bowl of freshly made hummus.

3. Enjoy your homemade hummus with warm whole wheat pita bread!

Stuffed Mushrooms with Spinach and Feta:

Ingredients:

- 20 large mushrooms, cleaned and stems removed
- 2 tablespoons olive oil
- 1 small onion, finely chopped
- 2 cloves garlic, minced
- 2 cups fresh spinach, chopped
- 1/2 cup feta cheese, crumbled
- 1/4 cup breadcrumbs
- Salt and pepper to taste
- Fresh parsley, chopped, for garnish

Instructions:

1. Preheat your oven to 375°F (190°C).

2. Clean the mushrooms and remove the stems. Finely chop the mushroom stems and set aside.

3. In a skillet, heat olive oil over medium heat. Add chopped onion and minced garlic, sautéing until softened.

4. Add the chopped mushroom stems to the skillet and cook for an additional 3-5 minutes.

5. Stir in the chopped spinach and cook until wilted. Season with salt and pepper to taste.

6. Remove the skillet from heat and let the mixture cool slightly.

7. In a bowl, combine the spinach and mushroom mixture with crumbled feta and breadcrumbs. Mix well.

8. Stuff each mushroom cap with the spinach and feta mixture, pressing it down slightly.

9. Arrange the stuffed mushrooms on a baking sheet.

10. Bake in the preheated oven for 15-20 minutes or until the mushrooms are tender and the tops are golden brown.

11. Garnish with freshly chopped parsley before serving.

12. Serve the stuffed mushrooms as an appetizer or a delightful party snack.

Brussels Sprouts Chips:

Ingredients:

- 1 pound Brussels sprouts, trimmed and halved
- 2 tablespoons olive oil
- Salt and pepper to taste
- Optional: Grated Parmesan cheese for topping

Instructions:

1. Preheat your oven to 400°F (200°C). Line a baking sheet with parchment paper.

2. Trim the Brussels sprouts and cut them in half. Remove any loose or damaged outer leaves.

3. In a bowl, toss the halved Brussels sprouts with olive oil, ensuring they are well coated.

4. Spread the Brussels sprouts evenly on the prepared baking sheet in a single layer.

5. Season with salt and pepper to taste. If desired, you can also sprinkle grated Parmesan cheese over the Brussels sprouts for added flavor.

6. Roast in the preheated oven for 20-25 minutes or until the edges are crispy and golden brown. Stir or shake the pan halfway through the cooking time for even crispiness.

7. Keep a close eye on them toward the end to prevent burning.

8. Remove from the oven and let them cool for a few minutes before serving.

9. Enjoy these Brussels sprouts chips as a tasty and nutritious snack or side dish.

Grilled Zucchini Roll-Ups:

Ingredients:

- 2 medium-sized zucchini
- Olive oil for brushing
- Salt and pepper to taste
- 1 cup ricotta cheese
- 1/4 cup grated Parmesan cheese
- 2 tablespoons fresh basil, chopped
- 1 clove garlic, minced
- Cherry tomatoes, for garnish (optional)
- Balsamic glaze, for drizzling (optional)

Instructions:

1. Preheat your grill or grill pan to medium-high heat.

2. Slice the zucchini lengthwise into thin strips using a mandoline slicer or a sharp knife. Aim for strips that are about 1/8 inch thick.

3. Brush the zucchini slices with olive oil on both sides and season with salt and pepper.

4. Grill the zucchini slices for 1-2 minutes per side or until they are slightly softened and have grill marks. Remove from the grill and let them cool.

5. In a bowl, mix together ricotta cheese, grated Parmesan, chopped fresh basil, and minced garlic. Season with salt and pepper to taste.

6. Place a spoonful of the ricotta mixture at one end of each zucchini strip.

7. Carefully roll up the zucchini, enclosing the ricotta filling. Repeat with the remaining strips.

8. Arrange the grilled zucchini roll-ups on a serving platter.

9. If desired, garnish with cherry tomatoes and drizzle with balsamic glaze for extra flavor.

10. Serve as an appetizer or a light, flavorful side dish.

Cucumber Avocado Salsa:

Ingredients:

- 2 medium-sized cucumbers, diced
- 2 ripe avocados, diced
- 1 cup cherry tomatoes, halved
- 1/4 cup red onion, finely chopped
- 1/4 cup fresh cilantro, chopped
- 1 jalapeño, seeded and finely chopped
- 2 cloves garlic, minced
- Juice of 2 limes
- 2 tablespoons extra virgin olive oil
- Salt and pepper to taste
- Optional: Dash of cayenne pepper for extra heat

Instructions:

1. In a large bowl, combine diced cucumbers, diced avocados, halved cherry tomatoes, finely chopped red onion, chopped fresh cilantro, and finely chopped jalapeño.
2. In a small bowl, whisk together minced garlic, lime juice, extra virgin olive oil, salt, and pepper. If you like it spicy, add a dash of cayenne pepper.
3. Pour the dressing over the cucumber and avocado mixture.
4. Gently toss the ingredients until well combined, ensuring the avocado is coated in the dressing to prevent browning.
5. Taste and adjust salt and pepper according to your preference.
6. Chill the cucumber avocado salsa in the refrigerator for at least 30 minutes to allow the flavors to meld.
7. Before serving, give it a final gentle stir.
8. Serve the cucumber avocado salsa as a refreshing side dish or a topping for grilled chicken, fish, or tacos.

Tomato Basil Mozzarella Skewers:

Ingredients:

- Cherry tomatoes
- Fresh mozzarella balls (bocconcini)
- Fresh basil leaves
- Balsamic glaze (store-bought or homemade)
- Extra virgin olive oil
- Salt and pepper to taste
- Wooden or cocktail skewers

Instructions:
1. Assemble the ingredients for easy access.
2. Rinse the cherry tomatoes and fresh basil leaves. Drain the fresh mozzarella balls if they are in liquid.
3. Take a wooden or cocktail skewer and thread a cherry tomato onto it, followed by a folded basil leaf, and then a mozzarella ball.

4. Repeat the process for the desired number of skewers.

5. Arrange the assembled Tomato Basil Mozzarella skewers on a serving platter.

6. Drizzle extra virgin olive oil over the skewers. Sprinkle with salt and pepper to taste.

7. Just before serving, generously drizzle balsamic glaze over the skewers. If you don't have balsamic glaze, you can reduce balsamic vinegar in a saucepan until it thickens.

8. Serve immediately as an elegant appetizer or a refreshing snack.

Whole Grain Crackers with Tuna Salad:

Ingredients:

For Tuna Salad:

- 1 can (5 oz) tuna, drained
- 1/4 cup mayonnaise
- 1 tablespoon Dijon mustard
- 2 tablespoons red onion, finely chopped
- 2 tablespoons celery, finely chopped
- 1 tablespoon fresh parsley, chopped
- Salt and pepper to taste
- Optional: Lemon juice for a fresh kick

For Serving:

- Whole grain crackers

Instructions:

1. In a bowl, combine drained tuna, mayonnaise, Dijon mustard, chopped red onion, chopped celery, and chopped fresh parsley.

2. Mix the ingredients until well combined. If desired, add a squeeze of lemon juice for a fresh flavor.

3. Season the tuna salad with salt and pepper to taste. Adjust the seasoning according to your preference.

4. Let the tuna salad chill in the refrigerator for at least 30 minutes to allow the flavors to meld.

5. Once the tuna salad is chilled, give it a final stir.

6. Arrange the whole grain crackers on a serving platter or plate.

7. Spoon the chilled tuna salad onto each cracker, spreading it evenly.

8. Garnish with additional chopped parsley or a sprinkle of black pepper if desired.

9. Serve the whole grain crackers with tuna salad as a wholesome and satisfying snack or light meal.

Kale and Berry Salad:

Ingredients:

For the Salad:

- 4 cups kale, stems removed and leaves chopped
- 1 cup mixed berries (strawberries, blueberries, raspberries)
- 1/2 cup sliced almonds, toasted
- 1/4 cup crumbled feta cheese (optional)

For the Dressing:

- 3 tablespoons extra virgin olive oil
- 1 tablespoon balsamic vinegar
- 1 teaspoon honey
- 1 teaspoon Dijon mustard
- Salt and pepper to taste

Instructions:

1. In a large salad bowl, place the chopped kale.
2. In a small dry skillet over medium heat, toast the sliced almonds until they are lightly browned. Keep a close eye on them to prevent burning. Once toasted, set them aside to cool.
3. Rinse the mixed berries and pat them dry with a paper towel.
4. Add the mixed berries and toasted sliced almonds to the bowl with kale.
5. If using, sprinkle crumbled feta cheese over the salad.
6. In a small bowl, whisk together extra virgin olive oil, balsamic vinegar, honey, Dijon mustard, salt, and pepper to make the dressing.
7. Pour the dressing over the salad ingredients.
8. Toss the salad gently until the ingredients are well coated with the dressing.

9. Let the kale and berry salad sit for a few minutes to allow the flavors to meld.

10. Serve the salad as a refreshing and nutritious side dish or add grilled chicken or salmon for a complete meal.

Salmon and Quinoa Salad:

Ingredients:

For the Salmon:

- 4 salmon fillets
- 2 tablespoons olive oil
- 1 teaspoon lemon zest
- 1 tablespoon lemon juice
- 1 teaspoon Dijon mustard
- Salt and pepper to taste

For the Quinoa:

- 1 cup quinoa, rinsed
- 2 cups water or broth
- Salt to taste

For the Salad:

- 4 cups mixed greens (spinach, arugula, or your choice)
- 1 cucumber, sliced
- 1 cup cherry tomatoes, halved
- 1/4 cup red onion, thinly sliced
- 1/4 cup feta cheese, crumbled

For the Lemon Vinaigrette:

- 3 tablespoons extra virgin olive oil
- 1 tablespoon lemon juice
- 1 teaspoon Dijon mustard
- 1 teaspoon honey
- Salt and pepper to taste

Instructions:

For the Salmon:

1. Preheat the oven to 400°F (200°C).
2. In a small bowl, whisk together olive oil, lemon zest, lemon juice, Dijon mustard, salt, and pepper.
3. Place the salmon fillets on a baking sheet lined with parchment paper. Brush the salmon with the prepared lemon-Dijon mixture.
4. Bake in the preheated oven for 12-15 minutes or until the salmon is cooked through and flakes easily with a fork.

For the Quinoa:

1. In a medium saucepan, combine quinoa, water or broth, and a pinch of salt.
2. Bring to a boil, then reduce the heat to low, cover, and simmer for 15-20 minutes or until the quinoa is cooked and water is absorbed.
3. Fluff the quinoa with a fork and let it cool slightly.

For the Lemon Vinaigrette:

1. In a small bowl, whisk together extra virgin olive oil, lemon juice, Dijon mustard, honey, salt, and pepper to make the vinaigrette.

Assembling the Salad:

1. In a large bowl, combine the cooked quinoa, mixed greens, sliced cucumber, cherry tomatoes, red onion, and crumbled feta cheese.
2. Drizzle the lemon vinaigrette over the salad and toss gently to coat.
3. Divide the salad among serving plates.
4. Place a baked salmon fillet on top of each salad.
5. Optionally, garnish with additional lemon wedges and fresh herbs.
6. Serve the Salmon and Quinoa Salad immediately as a wholesome and satisfying meal.

Mango Avocado Arugula Salad:

Ingredients:

For the Salad:

- 4 cups arugula, washed and dried
- 1 ripe mango, peeled, pitted, and diced
- 1 ripe avocado, peeled, pitted, and sliced
- 1/4 cup red onion, thinly sliced
- 1/4 cup crumbled feta cheese (optional)
- 2 tablespoons toasted pine nuts or sliced almonds (optional)

For the Dressing:

- 3 tablespoons extra virgin olive oil
- 1 tablespoon balsamic vinegar
- 1 teaspoon honey
- Salt and pepper to taste

Instructions:

1. In a large salad bowl, combine arugula, diced mango, sliced avocado, and thinly sliced red onion.
2. If using, add crumbled feta cheese for an extra layer of flavor.
3. In a small bowl, whisk together extra virgin olive oil, balsamic vinegar, honey, salt, and pepper to create the dressing.
4. Drizzle the dressing over the salad ingredients.
5. Toss the salad gently to ensure even coating of the dressing.
6. If desired, sprinkle toasted pine nuts or sliced almonds over the salad for added crunch.
7. Serve the Mango Avocado Arugula Salad immediately as a refreshing and vibrant side dish or a light meal.

Chickpea and Vegetable Mediterranean Salad:

Ingredients:

For the Salad:

- 1 can (15 oz) chickpeas, drained and rinsed

- 1 cup cherry tomatoes, halved
- 1 cucumber, diced
- 1 red bell pepper, diced
- 1/2 red onion, finely chopped
- 1/2 cup Kalamata olives, sliced
- 1/2 cup crumbled feta cheese
- 1/4 cup fresh parsley, chopped
- 1/4 cup fresh mint, chopped

For the Dressing:

- 3 tablespoons extra virgin olive oil
- 2 tablespoons red wine vinegar
- 1 clove garlic, minced
- 1 teaspoon dried oregano
- Salt and pepper to taste

Instructions:

1. In a large salad bowl, combine chickpeas, cherry tomatoes, diced cucumber, diced red bell pepper, finely chopped red onion, sliced Kalamata olives, crumbled feta cheese, fresh chopped parsley, and fresh chopped mint.
2. In a small bowl, whisk together extra virgin olive oil, red wine vinegar, minced garlic, dried oregano, salt, and pepper to create the dressing.
3. Pour the dressing over the salad ingredients.
4. Toss the salad gently to ensure even coating of the dressing.
5. Allow the salad to marinate for at least 15-20 minutes to enhance the flavors.
6. Serve the Chickpea and Vegetable Mediterranean Salad as a refreshing and wholesome side dish or a light meal.

Spinach and Pomegranate Salad:

Ingredients:

- 4 cups fresh baby spinach leaves

- 1 cup pomegranate arils
- 1/2 cup sliced almonds, toasted
- 1/4 cup crumbled feta cheese (optional)
- 1 tablespoon extra-virgin olive oil
- 1 tablespoon balsamic vinegar
- 1 teaspoon honey
- Salt and pepper to taste

Instructions:

1. Prepare the Spinach: Wash the baby spinach leaves thoroughly and pat them dry with a paper towel.

2. Toast the Almonds: In a dry skillet over medium heat, toast the sliced almonds until they turn golden brown. Be cautious not to burn them. Set aside to cool.

3. Seed the Pomegranate: Cut the pomegranate in half and gently tap the back with a wooden spoon to release the arils. Collect one cup of pomegranate arils and set aside.

4. Assemble the Salad: In a large bowl, combine the fresh baby spinach leaves, pomegranate arils, and toasted almonds. If desired, add crumbled feta cheese for extra flavor.

5. Prepare the Dressing: In a small bowl, whisk together the extra-virgin olive oil, balsamic vinegar, and honey. Season with salt and pepper to taste.

6. Drizzle and Toss: Pour the dressing over the salad and gently toss the ingredients until evenly coated.

7. Serve: Divide the salad into individual servings and enjoy this nutrient-rich, melanoma-friendly dish.

Grilled Chicken Caesar Salad:

Ingredients:

For the Grilled Chicken:

- 2 boneless, skinless chicken breasts

- 2 tablespoons olive oil
- 1 teaspoon dried oregano
- Salt and pepper to taste

For the Caesar Dressing:

- 1/2 cup mayonnaise
- 1/4 cup grated Parmesan cheese
- 2 tablespoons freshly squeezed lemon juice
- 1 tablespoon Dijon mustard
- 2 cloves garlic, minced
- Salt and pepper to taste

For the Salad:

- 1 large head of romaine lettuce, washed and chopped
- Croutons (store-bought or homemade)
- Additional grated Parmesan cheese for topping

Instructions:

1. Preheat the Grill: Preheat your grill to medium-high heat.
2. Prepare the Chicken: In a bowl, mix olive oil, dried oregano, salt, and pepper. Coat the chicken breasts with this mixture.
3. Grill the Chicken: Place the seasoned chicken breasts on the preheated grill. Grill for about 6-8 minutes per side or until the internal temperature reaches 165°F (74°C). Ensure the chicken is cooked through and has a nice char.
4. Make the Caesar Dressing: In a small bowl, whisk together mayonnaise, grated Parmesan cheese, lemon juice, Dijon mustard, minced garlic, salt, and pepper. Adjust the seasoning to taste.
5. Slice the Grilled Chicken: Allow the grilled chicken to rest for a few minutes, then slice it into thin strips.
6. Assemble the Salad: In a large bowl, combine the chopped romaine lettuce, croutons, and sliced grilled chicken.

7. Add the Dressing: Drizzle the Caesar dressing over the salad, tossing gently to coat the ingredients evenly.

8. Serve: Plate the salad, sprinkle with additional grated Parmesan cheese, and serve immediately.

Broccoli and Quinoa Salad:

Ingredients:

For the Salad:

- 1 cup quinoa, rinsed
- 2 cups broccoli florets, blanched
- 1/2 cup red bell pepper, diced
- 1/4 cup red onion, finely chopped
- 1/3 cup feta cheese, crumbled
- 1/4 cup sunflower seeds (optional, for crunch)
- Salt and pepper to taste

For the Dressing:

- 1/4 cup olive oil
- 2 tablespoons apple cider vinegar
- 1 tablespoon Dijon mustard
- 1 tablespoon honey
- 1 clove garlic, minced
- Salt and pepper to taste

Instructions:

1. Cook the Quinoa: In a medium saucepan, combine 2 cups of water with the rinsed quinoa. Bring to a boil, then reduce heat, cover, and simmer for about 15 minutes or until quinoa is cooked and water is absorbed. Fluff with a fork and let it cool.

2. Blanch the Broccoli: Bring a pot of water to boil. Add broccoli florets and cook for 2-3 minutes until they turn bright green. Quickly transfer the broccoli to a bowl of ice water to stop the cooking process. Drain and set aside.

3. Prepare Vegetables: In a large bowl, combine the cooked quinoa, blanched broccoli, diced red bell pepper, chopped red onion, feta cheese, and sunflower seeds.

4. Make the Dressing: In a small bowl, whisk together olive oil, apple cider vinegar, Dijon mustard, honey, minced garlic, salt, and pepper.

5. Combine and Toss: Pour the dressing over the salad ingredients. Toss everything together until well coated with the dressing.

6. Season to Taste: Adjust salt and pepper as needed.

7. Chill and Serve: Refrigerate the salad for at least 30 minutes before serving to let the flavors meld. Serve chilled.

Watermelon and Feta Salad:

Ingredients:

- 4 cups cubed seedless watermelon
- 1 cup crumbled feta cheese
- 1/2 cup fresh mint leaves, chopped
- 1/4 cup red onion, thinly sliced
- 2 tablespoons extra-virgin olive oil
- 1 tablespoon balsamic glaze
- Salt and pepper to taste

Instructions:

1. Prepare the Watermelon: Cut the watermelon into bite-sized cubes, removing seeds if necessary. Place the watermelon cubes in a large mixing bowl.

2. Add Feta and Onion: Crumble the feta cheese over the watermelon. Add thinly sliced red onion to the bowl.

3. Toss with Mint: Sprinkle the chopped fresh mint leaves over the ingredients in the bowl.

4. Drizzle with Olive Oil: Drizzle extra-virgin olive oil over the salad for added richness.

5. Season and Toss: Season the salad with salt and pepper to taste. Gently toss all the ingredients together to ensure an even distribution of flavors.

6. Drizzle with Balsamic Glaze: Just before serving, drizzle balsamic glaze over the salad for a sweet and tangy finish.

7. Chill (Optional): For a refreshing touch, you can chill the salad in the refrigerator for about 30 minutes before serving.

8. Serve: Plate the watermelon and feta salad and enjoy this delightful combination of sweet and savory flavors.

Tuna and Bean Salad:

Ingredients:

- 2 cans (15 oz each) cannellini beans, drained and rinsed
- 2 cans (5 oz each) tuna in olive oil, drained
- 1 cup cherry tomatoes, halved
- 1/2 cup red onion, finely chopped
- 1/4 cup fresh parsley, chopped
- 1/4 cup Kalamata olives, sliced
- 2 tablespoons capers, drained
- 3 tablespoons extra-virgin olive oil
- 2 tablespoons red wine vinegar
- 1 teaspoon Dijon mustard
- Salt and pepper to taste
- Lemon wedges for serving

Instructions:

1. Prepare the Beans: In a large bowl, combine the cannellini beans, drained tuna, halved cherry tomatoes, chopped red onion, fresh parsley, sliced Kalamata olives, and capers.

2. Make the Dressing: In a small bowl, whisk together the extra-virgin olive oil, red wine vinegar, Dijon mustard, salt, and pepper. Adjust the seasoning to taste.

3. Combine and Toss: Pour the dressing over the bean and tuna mixture. Gently toss the ingredients until well coated with the dressing.

4. Chill (Optional): Allow the salad to chill in the refrigerator for about 15-30 minutes to let the flavors meld.

5. Serve: Portion the tuna and bean salad onto plates. Serve with lemon wedges on the side for an extra burst of freshness.

Cabbage and Apple Slaw:

Ingredients:

- 4 cups shredded green cabbage
- 2 medium-sized apples, julienned
- 1/2 cup shredded carrots
- 1/4 cup red onion, thinly sliced
- 1/2 cup plain Greek yogurt
- 2 tablespoons mayonnaise
- 2 tablespoons apple cider vinegar
- 1 tablespoon honey
- 1 teaspoon Dijon mustard
- Salt and pepper to taste
- 1/4 cup chopped fresh parsley (optional, for garnish)

Instructions:

1. Prepare the Vegetables: In a large bowl, combine the shredded green cabbage, julienned apples, shredded carrots, and thinly sliced red onion.

2. Make the Dressing: In a separate bowl, whisk together the Greek yogurt, mayonnaise, apple cider vinegar, honey, Dijon mustard, salt, and pepper. Adjust the seasoning to taste.

3. Combine and Toss: Pour the dressing over the cabbage and apple mixture. Toss the ingredients until the slaw is evenly coated with the dressing.

4. Chill (Optional): Allow the slaw to chill in the refrigerator for at least 30 minutes before serving. This enhances the flavors and crispness.

5. Garnish (Optional): Just before serving, sprinkle chopped fresh parsley over the slaw for a burst of color and added freshness.

6. Serve: Portion the cabbage and apple slaw onto plates or into bowls. It makes a refreshing side dish for various meals.

Quinoa and Mango Black Bean Salad:

Ingredients:

- 1 cup quinoa, rinsed
- 2 cups water or vegetable broth
- 1 can (15 oz) black beans, drained and rinsed
- 1 ripe mango, peeled and diced
- 1 red bell pepper, diced
- 1/2 red onion, finely chopped
- 1/4 cup fresh cilantro, chopped
- Juice of 2 limes
- 2 tablespoons extra-virgin olive oil
- 1 teaspoon ground cumin
- Salt and pepper to taste
- Optional: Avocado slices for garnish

Instructions:

1. Cook the Quinoa: In a medium saucepan, combine quinoa and water or vegetable broth. Bring to a boil, then reduce heat, cover, and simmer for about 15 minutes or until quinoa is cooked and liquid is absorbed. Fluff with a fork and let it cool.

2. Prepare the Black Beans: Drain and rinse the black beans under cold water.

3. Combine Ingredients: In a large bowl, mix the cooked quinoa, black beans, diced mango, diced red bell pepper, finely chopped red onion, and chopped cilantro.

4. Make the Dressing: In a small bowl, whisk together lime juice, extra-virgin olive oil, ground cumin, salt, and pepper.

5. Toss with Dressing: Pour the dressing over the quinoa mixture. Toss everything together until well combined and evenly coated with the dressing.

6. Chill (Optional): Refrigerate the salad for about 30 minutes to let the flavors meld. This step enhances the taste.

7. Garnish (Optional): Before serving, garnish with avocado slices for extra creaminess.

8. Serve: Portion the quinoa and mango black bean salad onto plates and enjoy this nutritious and vibrant dish.

Avocado and Shrimp Salad:

Ingredients:

- 1 pound large shrimp, peeled and deveined
- 2 avocados, diced
- 1 cup cherry tomatoes, halved
- 1/4 cup red onion, finely chopped
- 1/4 cup fresh cilantro, chopped
- 1 jalapeño, seeded and finely chopped (optional, for heat)
- 2 tablespoons extra-virgin olive oil
- 2 tablespoons lime juice
- 1 clove garlic, minced
- Salt and pepper to taste
- Mixed salad greens for serving

Instructions:

1. Cook the Shrimp: In a large pot of boiling salted water, cook the shrimp for 2-3 minutes or until they turn pink and opaque. Drain and let them cool.

2. Prepare the Salad Base: In a large bowl, combine diced avocados, halved cherry tomatoes, finely chopped red onion, chopped cilantro, and, if desired, finely chopped jalapeño for a bit of heat.

3. Make the Dressing: In a small bowl, whisk together extra-virgin olive oil, lime juice, minced garlic, salt, and pepper.

4. Combine and Toss: Add the cooked shrimp to the salad base. Pour the dressing over the ingredients and gently toss everything together until well coated.

5. Chill (Optional): Allow the salad to chill in the refrigerator for about 15-30 minutes before serving. This helps the flavors meld.

6. Serve on Greens: Serve the avocado and shrimp salad over a bed of mixed salad greens for a complete and satisfying meal.

7. Garnish (Optional): Garnish with additional cilantro or a lime wedge before serving.

Lentil and Vegetable Salad:

Ingredients:

- 1 cup dried green or brown lentils, rinsed
- 3 cups water or vegetable broth
- 1 cup cherry tomatoes, halved
- 1 cucumber, diced
- 1 red bell pepper, diced
- 1/2 red onion, finely chopped
- 1/4 cup fresh parsley, chopped
- 1/4 cup feta cheese, crumbled (optional)
- 3 tablespoons extra-virgin olive oil
- 2 tablespoons red wine vinegar
- 1 teaspoon Dijon mustard
- 1 clove garlic, minced
- Salt and pepper to taste

Instructions:

1. Cook the Lentils: In a medium saucepan, combine the lentils and water or vegetable broth. Bring to a boil, then reduce heat, cover, and simmer for about 20-25 minutes or until lentils are tender but still hold their shape. Drain any excess liquid and let the lentils cool.

2. Prepare the Vegetables: In a large bowl, combine the cooked lentils, halved cherry tomatoes, diced cucumber, diced red bell pepper, finely chopped red onion, and chopped fresh parsley.

3. Make the Dressing: In a small bowl, whisk together extra-virgin olive oil, red wine vinegar, Dijon mustard, minced garlic, salt, and pepper.

4. Combine and Toss: Pour the dressing over the lentil and vegetable mixture. Gently toss everything together until well coated with the dressing.

5. Add Feta (Optional): If desired, sprinkle crumbled feta cheese over the salad for extra flavor.

6. Chill (Optional): Refrigerate the lentil and vegetable salad for about 30 minutes before serving. This step enhances the flavors.

7. Serve: Portion the salad onto plates or into bowls. It can be enjoyed as a light and nutritious main or side dish.

DESSERT:

Mixed Berry Parfait:

Ingredients:

- 2 cups mixed berries (strawberries, blueberries, raspberries)
- 2 tablespoons honey or maple syrup
- 2 cups Greek yogurt (or yogurt of your choice)
- 1 teaspoon vanilla extract
- 1 cup granola
- Fresh mint leaves for garnish (optional)

Instructions:

1. Prepare the Berries: Wash and hull strawberries, then slice them into bite-sized pieces. If using other berries, rinse them as well.

2. Sweeten the Berries: In a bowl, combine the mixed berries with honey or maple syrup. Toss gently to coat the berries, allowing them to macerate and release some natural juices.

3. Flavor the Yogurt: In another bowl, mix Greek yogurt with vanilla extract. Stir well to combine, creating a flavorful yogurt base.

4. Assemble the Parfaits: In serving glasses or bowls, layer the components. Begin with a spoonful of the sweetened mixed berries, followed by a layer of vanilla-flavored yogurt, and then a sprinkle of granola.

5. Repeat Layers: Continue layering until you reach the top of the glass, finishing with a final dollop of yogurt.

6. Top with Granola and Berries: Sprinkle additional granola over the top layer of yogurt and garnish with a few fresh berries for an appealing presentation.

7. Garnish (Optional): If desired, garnish the parfait with fresh mint leaves for a burst of freshness.

8. Serve Immediately: Enjoy the mixed berry parfait immediately for the best texture and flavor contrast.

Dark Chocolate-Dipped Strawberries:

Ingredients:

- 1 pound fresh strawberries, washed and dried
- 8 ounces dark chocolate (at least 70% cocoa), chopped
- 1 tablespoon coconut oil or vegetable oil (optional, for smoothness)
- Toppings (optional): Chopped nuts, shredded coconut, sprinkles

Instructions:

1. Prepare Strawberries: Wash and thoroughly dry the strawberries. Make sure they are completely dry to help the chocolate adhere better.

2. Melt the Dark Chocolate: In a heatproof bowl, melt the dark chocolate. You can do this using a double boiler or by microwaving in 20-30 second intervals, stirring between each interval. If the chocolate is too thick, you can add coconut oil or vegetable oil to achieve a smoother consistency.

3. Dip the Strawberries: Holding each strawberry by the stem, dip it into the melted chocolate, covering about two-thirds of the berry. Allow excess chocolate to drip back into the bowl.

4. Set on Parchment Paper: Place the chocolate-dipped strawberries on a parchment paper-lined tray or plate. This prevents them from sticking and makes for easy cleanup.

5. Add Toppings (Optional): While the chocolate is still wet, you can sprinkle your preferred toppings such as chopped nuts, shredded coconut, or sprinkles over the dipped part of the strawberries.

6. Cool and Set: Allow the chocolate-dipped strawberries to cool and set. You can speed up this process by placing them in the refrigerator for about 15-20 minutes.

7. Serve: Once the chocolate is fully set, transfer the dark chocolate-dipped strawberries to a serving plate. They are now ready to be enjoyed.

Chia Seed Pudding with Mango:

Ingredients:

- 1/4 cup chia seeds
- 1 cup almond milk (or any milk of your choice)
- 1 tablespoon maple syrup or honey
- 1/2 teaspoon vanilla extract
- 1 ripe mango, peeled and diced
- Optional toppings: Sliced almonds, shredded coconut, additional diced mango

Instructions:

1. Mix Chia Seed Pudding Base:

o   In a bowl, combine chia seeds, almond milk, maple syrup or honey, and vanilla extract.

o   Whisk the ingredients together thoroughly to ensure the chia seeds are well distributed.

2. Refrigerate Overnight:

o   Cover the bowl and refrigerate the chia seed mixture for at least 4 hours, or preferably overnight. This allows the chia seeds to absorb the liquid and create a pudding-like consistency.

3. Stir Before Serving:

o   Before serving, give the chia seed pudding a good stir to break up any clumps that may have formed during the refrigeration process.

4. Assemble with Mango:

o   In serving glasses or bowls, layer the chia seed pudding with diced mango. You can create alternating layers or simply top the pudding with a generous serving of mango.

5. Add Toppings:

o   If desired, sprinkle sliced almonds, shredded coconut, or additional diced mango on top for added texture and flavor.

6. Serve Chilled:

o   Serve the Chia Seed Pudding with Mango immediately, or refrigerate until ready to enjoy. The pudding is best when served chilled.

Baked Apples with Cinnamon:

Ingredients:

- 4 large apples (such as Honeycrisp or Granny Smith)
- 1/4 cup brown sugar
- 1 teaspoon ground cinnamon
- 1/4 teaspoon ground nutmeg
- 2 tablespoons unsalted butter, cut into small pieces

- 1/2 cup chopped nuts (walnuts or pecans, optional)
- 1/2 cup raisins or dried cranberries (optional)
- Vanilla ice cream or whipped cream for serving (optional)

Instructions:

1. Preheat the Oven:
   - Preheat your oven to 375°F (190°C).
2. Prepare the Apples:
   - Wash and core the apples, leaving the bottoms intact. You can use an apple corer or a knife to remove the cores, creating a well for the filling.
3. Mix the Filling:
   - In a small bowl, combine brown sugar, ground cinnamon, and ground nutmeg. Mix well.
4. Fill the Apples:
   - Place the cored apples in a baking dish. Fill each apple with the brown sugar and cinnamon mixture, distributing it evenly among the apples.
5. Add Butter and Extras:
   - Place small pieces of butter on top of each filled apple. If using, sprinkle chopped nuts and raisins or dried cranberries over the apples.
6. Bake:
   - Bake in the preheated oven for approximately 30-40 minutes or until the apples are tender but not mushy. The baking time may vary depending on the size and type of apples you use.
7. Baste (Optional):
   - If desired, baste the apples with the juices from the baking dish halfway through the baking time to enhance flavor.
8. Serve:
   - Remove the baked apples from the oven. Let them cool for a few minutes before serving. Optionally, serve with a scoop of vanilla ice cream or a dollop of whipped cream for a delightful treat.

Frozen Banana Bites:

Ingredients:

- 2 large bananas, peeled and sliced into rounds
- 1/2 cup chocolate chips (dark, milk, or white chocolate)
- 1 tablespoon coconut oil
- Toppings of your choice: Chopped nuts, shredded coconut, sprinkles

Instructions:

1. Prepare Banana Slices:
   - Slice the bananas into rounds, about 1/2 inch thick. Place the banana slices on a parchment paper-lined tray or plate.
2. Freeze Banana Slices:
   - Freeze the banana slices for at least 30 minutes. This step helps the chocolate coating adhere better.
3. Melt Chocolate:
   - In a microwave-safe bowl or using a double boiler, melt the chocolate chips and coconut oil together. Stir until smooth.
4. Dip Banana Slices:
   - Take the frozen banana slices and dip each one into the melted chocolate, ensuring that each side is coated. Allow excess chocolate to drip back into the bowl.
5. Add Toppings:
   - While the chocolate is still wet, sprinkle your desired toppings over the banana slices. You can use chopped nuts, shredded coconut, or sprinkles for added texture and flavor.
6. Freeze Again:
   - Place the chocolate-coated banana slices back on the parchment paper-lined tray and freeze for an additional 1-2 hours or until the chocolate is fully set.
7. Serve:

o Once the frozen banana bites are completely set, transfer them to a serving plate. They are now ready to be enjoyed.

Coconut and Berry Sorbet:

Ingredients:

- 2 cups mixed berries (strawberries, blueberries, raspberries)
- 1 can (14 oz) coconut milk (full-fat for creamier texture)
- 1/3 cup honey or maple syrup (adjust to taste)
- 1 teaspoon vanilla extract
- Zest and juice of 1 lime
- Pinch of salt

Instructions:

1. Prepare the Berries:
   - Wash the berries and pat them dry. If using strawberries, hull and slice them into smaller pieces.
2. Blend the Ingredients:
   - In a blender, combine the mixed berries, coconut milk, honey or maple syrup, vanilla extract, lime zest, lime juice, and a pinch of salt. Blend until smooth.
3. Taste and Adjust:
   - Taste the mixture and adjust the sweetness if needed by adding more honey or maple syrup. Blend again to combine.
4. Strain (Optional):
   - If you prefer a smoother sorbet, you can strain the mixture through a fine-mesh sieve to remove berry seeds. This step is optional.
5. Chill the Mixture:
   - Refrigerate the blended mixture for at least 2 hours to chill thoroughly.
6. Churn in Ice Cream Maker:

o Pour the chilled mixture into an ice cream maker and churn according to the manufacturer's instructions until it reaches a sorbet-like consistency.

7. Transfer to Container:

   o Transfer the churned sorbet into a lidded container and freeze for an additional 2-4 hours, or until it firms up.

8. Serve:

   o Scoop the Coconut and Berry Sorbet into bowls or cones. Garnish with fresh berries or a sprinkle of shredded coconut if desired.

Almond and Blueberry Energy Bites:

Ingredients:

- 1 cup rolled oats
- 1/2 cup almond butter
- 1/3 cup honey or maple syrup
- 1/2 cup almond meal
- 1/2 cup dried blueberries
- 1/4 cup ground flaxseeds
- 1 teaspoon vanilla extract
- Pinch of salt
- Optional: Shredded coconut for coating

Instructions:

1. Combine Dry Ingredients:

   o In a large bowl, mix together rolled oats, almond meal, dried blueberries, ground flaxseeds, and a pinch of salt.

2. Add Wet Ingredients:

   o Add almond butter, honey or maple syrup, and vanilla extract to the dry ingredients. Stir well to combine.

3. Chill the Mixture:

- o Place the mixture in the refrigerator for about 30 minutes. Chilling makes it easier to handle and shape into bites.

4. Shape into Bites:
   - o After chilling, take small portions of the mixture and roll them into bite-sized balls using your hands. If desired, roll each bite in shredded coconut for an extra layer of flavor.

5. Set in the Fridge:
   - o Place the almond and blueberry energy bites on a parchment paper-lined tray or plate and refrigerate for at least 1 hour to firm up.

6. Store:
   - o Once the energy bites are set, transfer them to an airtight container and store in the refrigerator for freshness.

7. Enjoy:
   - o These energy bites can be enjoyed as a quick snack or a pre-workout boost. Grab one or two whenever you need a burst of energy.

Pineapple Mint Sorbet:

Ingredients:

- 4 cups fresh pineapple chunks (about 1 medium-sized pineapple)
- 1/2 cup fresh mint leaves, packed
- 1/2 cup granulated sugar
- 1/4 cup water
- 2 tablespoons fresh lime juice
- Optional: Mint leaves for garnish

Instructions:

1. Prepare Pineapple:
   - o Peel and core the pineapple, then cut it into chunks.

2. Make Mint Simple Syrup:

o In a small saucepan, combine sugar, water, and fresh mint leaves. Heat over medium heat, stirring until the sugar dissolves. Once the mixture comes to a simmer, let it simmer for an additional 2-3 minutes. Remove from heat and let it cool. Strain to remove mint leaves, leaving you with mint-infused simple syrup.

3. Blend Pineapple and Mint Syrup:

   o In a blender, combine fresh pineapple chunks, mint-infused simple syrup, and fresh lime juice. Blend until smooth.

4. Strain (Optional):

   o For a smoother sorbet, you can strain the mixture through a fine-mesh sieve to remove any pulp. This step is optional.

5. Chill the Mixture:

   o Refrigerate the blended mixture for at least 2 hours to chill thoroughly.

6. Churn in Ice Cream Maker:

   o Pour the chilled mixture into an ice cream maker and churn according to the manufacturer's instructions until it reaches a sorbet-like consistency.

7. Transfer to Container:

   o Transfer the churned sorbet into a lidded container and freeze for an additional 2-4 hours, or until it firms up.

8. Serve:

   o Scoop the Pineapple Mint Sorbet into bowls or cones. Garnish with fresh mint leaves if desired.

Avocado Chocolate Mousse:

Ingredients:

- 2 ripe avocados, peeled and pitted
- 1/2 cup cocoa powder (unsweetened)
- 1/2 cup maple syrup or agave nectar
- 1/3 cup coconut milk (or any milk of your choice)

- 1 teaspoon vanilla extract
- Pinch of salt
- Optional toppings: Fresh berries, chopped nuts, or whipped cream

Instructions:

1. Blend Avocado:
   - In a food processor or blender, combine the ripe avocados, cocoa powder, maple syrup or agave nectar, coconut milk, vanilla extract, and a pinch of salt.
2. Blend Until Smooth:
   - Blend the ingredients until you achieve a smooth and creamy consistency. Scrape down the sides of the blender or food processor as needed.
3. Taste and Adjust:
   - Taste the mixture and adjust the sweetness if necessary by adding more maple syrup or agave nectar. Blend again to combine.
4. Chill (Optional):
   - For a thicker and chilled mousse, you can refrigerate the mixture for at least 30 minutes before serving.
5. Serve:
   - Spoon the Avocado Chocolate Mousse into serving glasses or bowls.
6. Add Toppings:
   - Garnish with your favorite toppings such as fresh berries, chopped nuts, or a dollop of whipped cream.
7. Enjoy:
   - Serve immediately and enjoy this rich and indulgent Avocado Chocolate Mousse.

Baked Peaches with Almond Crumble:

Ingredients:

- 4 ripe peaches, halved and pitted

- 2 tablespoons lemon juice
- 2 tablespoons brown sugar
- 1/2 teaspoon ground cinnamon

For the Almond Crumble:

- 1/2 cup almond flour
- 1/4 cup rolled oats
- 2 tablespoons almond butter
- 2 tablespoons maple syrup or honey
- 1/2 teaspoon vanilla extract
- Pinch of salt

Instructions:

1. Preheat the Oven:
   - Preheat your oven to 375°F (190°C).
2. Prepare the Peaches:
   - Halve the peaches and remove the pits. Place the peach halves in a baking dish.
3. Lemon Drizzle:
   - Drizzle lemon juice over the peach halves to enhance flavor and prevent browning.
4. Sprinkle with Sugar and Cinnamon:
   - Sprinkle brown sugar and ground cinnamon over the peach halves, distributing them evenly.
5. Make the Almond Crumble:
   - In a bowl, combine almond flour, rolled oats, almond butter, maple syrup or honey, vanilla extract, and a pinch of salt. Mix until the ingredients form a crumbly texture.
6. Top the Peaches:
   - Spoon the almond crumble mixture onto each peach half, pressing it gently to adhere.

7. Bake:
   - Bake in the preheated oven for about 20-25 minutes or until the peaches are tender, and the almond crumble is golden brown.
8. Serve Warm:
   - Remove from the oven and let it cool slightly. Serve the baked peaches warm.
9. Optional: Garnish:
   - Optionally, garnish with a sprinkle of additional cinnamon, a drizzle of honey, or a scoop of vanilla ice cream for added indulgence.

Yogurt and Berry Popsicles:

Ingredients:

- 1 cup Greek yogurt (or regular yogurt)
- 2 tablespoons honey or maple syrup (adjust to taste)
- 1 teaspoon vanilla extract
- 1 cup mixed berries (strawberries, blueberries, raspberries)
- Popsicle molds

Instructions:

1. Prepare Yogurt Mixture:
   - In a bowl, mix Greek yogurt, honey or maple syrup, and vanilla extract. Stir until well combined. Taste and adjust sweetness if needed.
2. Prepare Berries:
   - Wash and slice the strawberries. If using larger berries, you can halve or quarter them for easier handling.
3. Layer Yogurt and Berries:
   - Begin by spooning a layer of the yogurt mixture into each popsicle mold, filling it about one-third of the way.
4. Add Berries:

- o Drop a few slices of berries into each mold. You can gently press them down to distribute them evenly.

5. Repeat Layers:
   - o Continue layering with more yogurt, then berries, until the molds are almost full. Ensure you finish with a layer of yogurt on top.

6. Insert Popsicle Sticks:
   - o Place the popsicle sticks into the molds. Make sure they are centered, and they go down into the yogurt mixture.

7. Freeze:
   - o Place the popsicle molds in the freezer and let them freeze for at least 4-6 hours or until completely solid.

8. Unmold Popsicles:
   - o Once frozen, remove the popsicle molds from the freezer. To unmold, run the molds under warm water for a few seconds to loosen the popsicles.

Lemon Sorbet with Basil:

Ingredients:

- 1 cup fresh lemon juice (about 6-8 lemons)
- 1 cup granulated sugar
- 2 cups water
- Zest of 2 lemons
- 1/4 cup fresh basil leaves, chopped
- Optional: Basil leaves for garnish

Instructions:

1. Prepare Lemon Juice:
   - o Squeeze enough lemons to obtain 1 cup of fresh lemon juice. This is typically around 6-8 lemons depending on their size and juiciness.

2. Make Simple Syrup:

o In a saucepan, combine granulated sugar and water. Heat over medium heat, stirring until the sugar dissolves completely. Bring the mixture to a gentle simmer, then remove from heat.

3. Infuse with Lemon Zest:

   o Add the lemon zest to the simple syrup, stirring to combine. Let it steep for about 15-20 minutes to infuse the syrup with lemon flavor. Allow it to cool.

4. Strain (Optional):

   o If you prefer a smoother sorbet, you can strain the simple syrup to remove the lemon zest. This step is optional.

5. Combine Lemon Juice and Basil:

   o In a bowl, combine the fresh lemon juice with the chopped fresh basil. This will infuse the lemon juice with the aromatic essence of basil.

6. Mix Lemon Juice and Simple Syrup:

   o Strain the lemon-basil mixture into the cooled simple syrup. Stir well to combine.

7. Chill the Mixture:

   o Refrigerate the lemon-basil mixture for at least 2 hours to chill thoroughly.

8. Churn in Ice Cream Maker:

   o Pour the chilled mixture into an ice cream maker and churn according to the manufacturer's instructions until it reaches a sorbet-like consistency.

9. Transfer to Container:

   o Transfer the churned sorbet into a lidded container and freeze for an additional 2-4 hours, or until it firms up.

10. Serve:

   o Scoop the Lemon Sorbet with Basil into bowls or cones. Garnish with fresh basil leaves if desired.

Walnut and Date Bliss Balls

Ingredients:

- 1 cup pitted dates
- 1 cup walnuts
- 1/4 cup unsweetened shredded coconut
- 1 tablespoon chia seeds (optional)
- 1 teaspoon vanilla extract
- Pinch of salt
- Additional shredded coconut for rolling (optional)

Instructions:

1. Prepare Dates:
   - If the dates are not already pitted, remove the pits. You can soften them by soaking in warm water for 10-15 minutes if they are very dry.
2. Blend Dates and Walnuts:
   - In a food processor, combine the pitted dates and walnuts. Pulse until they are broken down into small pieces and begin to form a sticky mixture.
3. Add Coconut and Chia Seeds:
   - Add the unsweetened shredded coconut, chia seeds (if using), vanilla extract, and a pinch of salt to the date and walnut mixture.
4. Blend Until Combined:
   - Continue pulsing the ingredients in the food processor until the mixture comes together into a sticky, uniform consistency. You should be able to press it between your fingers and it holds together.
5. Shape into Balls:
   - Take small portions of the mixture and roll it between your palms to form bite-sized bliss balls.
6. Optional: Roll in Coconut:
   - If desired, roll the bliss balls in additional shredded coconut for a coating.
7. Chill (Optional):
   - For a firmer texture and to allow flavors to meld, you can refrigerate the bliss balls for about 30 minutes before serving.
8. Serve:
   - Enjoy these Walnut and Date Bliss Balls as a healthy snack or a quick energy boost.

CHAPTER 8: SMOOTHIES AND BEVERAGES TO SUPPORT HEALING

Berry Blast Smoothie:

Ingredients:

- 1 cup mixed berries (strawberries, blueberries, raspberries)
- 1/2 banana, frozen
- 1/2 cup Greek yogurt
- 1/2 cup almond milk (or any milk of your choice)
- 1 tablespoon honey or maple syrup (optional, for added sweetness)
- 1/2 cup ice cubes
- Optional: Chia seeds or flaxseeds for extra nutrition

Instructions:

1. Prepare Ingredients:
   - Wash the berries and remove any stems. Peel and slice the banana before freezing.
2. Combine in Blender:
   - In a blender, combine the mixed berries, frozen banana slices, Greek yogurt, almond milk, and honey or maple syrup if using.
3. Add Ice Cubes:
   - Toss in the ice cubes to add a refreshing and chilled element to the smoothie.
4. Optional: Include Seeds:
   - For added nutrition, you can include a tablespoon of chia seeds or flaxseeds into the blender.
5. Blend Until Smooth:

o Blend all the ingredients until smooth and creamy. If the consistency is too thick, you can add more almond milk in small increments until it reaches your desired thickness.

6. Taste and Adjust:
   o Taste the smoothie and adjust the sweetness if needed by adding more honey or maple syrup.

7. Pour and Serve:
   o Pour the Berry Blast Smoothie into glasses and serve immediately.

8. Garnish (Optional):
   o If you like, garnish the smoothie with a few whole berries on top for a decorative touch.

9. Enjoy:
   o Sip and enjoy this refreshing Berry Blast Smoothie for a burst of fruity goodness. It's perfect for breakfast, a snack, or a post-workout pick-me-up.

Green Goddess Smoothie:

Ingredients:

- 1 cup fresh spinach leaves
- 1/2 cucumber, peeled and sliced
- 1/2 avocado, pitted and peeled
- 1/2 banana, frozen
- 1/2 cup Greek yogurt
- 1/2 cup coconut water (or regular water)
- 1 tablespoon chia seeds
- Fresh mint leaves (optional, for added freshness)
- Ice cubes (optional, for extra chill)
- Honey or maple syrup (optional, for added sweetness)

Instructions:

1. Prepare Ingredients:

- Wash the spinach leaves and cucumber. Peel and slice the cucumber. Pit and peel the avocado. Slice the banana before freezing.

2. Combine in Blender:
   - In a blender, combine fresh spinach leaves, cucumber slices, avocado, frozen banana slices, Greek yogurt, chia seeds, and coconut water.

3. Add Fresh Mint (Optional):
   - For an extra burst of freshness, add a few fresh mint leaves to the blender.

4. Include Ice Cubes (Optional):
   - If you prefer a colder smoothie, toss in a handful of ice cubes.

5. Blend Until Smooth:
   - Blend all the ingredients until smooth and creamy. If the consistency is too thick, you can add more coconut water or regular water in small increments until it reaches your desired thickness.

6. Optional Sweetening:
   - Taste the Green Goddess Smoothie and add honey or maple syrup if you desire additional sweetness. Blend again to combine.

7. Pour and Serve:
   - Pour the smoothie into glasses and serve immediately.

8. Garnish (Optional):
   - Optionally, garnish the Green Goddess Smoothie with a slice of cucumber or a sprinkle of chia seeds for visual appeal.

9. Enjoy:
   - Sip and enjoy this nutrient-packed Green Goddess Smoothie for a refreshing and wholesome start to your day or as a healthy snack.

Turmeric Mango Smoothie:

Ingredients:

- 1 cup frozen mango chunks
- 1/2 banana, frozen

- 1 cup coconut milk (or any milk of your choice)
- 1/2 teaspoon ground turmeric
- 1/2 teaspoon ground ginger
- 1 tablespoon chia seeds
- 1 tablespoon honey or maple syrup (optional, for added sweetness)
- Ice cubes (optional, for extra chill)

Instructions:

1. Prepare Ingredients:
   - Peel and slice the banana before freezing. If using fresh mango, you can freeze mango chunks in advance.
2. Combine in Blender:
   - In a blender, combine the frozen mango chunks, frozen banana slices, coconut milk, ground turmeric, ground ginger, and chia seeds.
3. Add Sweetener (Optional):
   - If you prefer a sweeter smoothie, add honey or maple syrup to the blender.
4. Include Ice Cubes (Optional):
   - For an extra chilly smoothie, toss in a handful of ice cubes.
5. Blend Until Smooth:
   - Blend all the ingredients until smooth and creamy. If the consistency is too thick, you can add more coconut milk or water in small increments until it reaches your desired thickness.
6. Taste and Adjust:
   - Taste the Turmeric Mango Smoothie and adjust the sweetness or spice level according to your preference.
7. Pour and Serve:
   - Pour the smoothie into glasses and serve immediately.
8. Garnish (Optional):
   - Optionally, garnish the Turmeric Mango Smoothie with a sprinkle of chia seeds or a slice of fresh mango for a decorative touch.

Protein-Packed Almond Butter Banana Smoothie:

Ingredients:

- 1 banana, frozen
- 1 cup almond milk (or any milk of your choice)
- 2 tablespoons almond butter
- 1 scoop vanilla protein powder
- 1 tablespoon chia seeds
- 1/2 teaspoon cinnamon
- Ice cubes (optional, for extra chill)
- Honey or maple syrup (optional, for added sweetness)

Instructions:

1. Prepare Ingredients:
   - Peel and slice the banana before freezing.
2. Combine in Blender:
   - In a blender, combine the frozen banana slices, almond milk, almond butter, vanilla protein powder, chia seeds, and cinnamon.
3. Add Sweetener (Optional):
   - If you prefer a sweeter smoothie, add honey or maple syrup to the blender.
4. Include Ice Cubes (Optional):
   - For an extra cold and refreshing smoothie, add a handful of ice cubes.
5. Blend Until Smooth:
   - Blend all the ingredients until smooth and creamy. If the consistency is too thick, you can add more almond milk or water in small increments until it reaches your desired thickness.
6. Taste and Adjust:
   - Taste the smoothie and adjust the sweetness or thickness according to your preference.
7. Pour and Serve:

o Pour the Protein-Packed Almond Butter Banana Smoothie into glasses and serve immediately.

Citrus Sunrise Smoothie:

Ingredients:

- 1 orange, peeled and segmented
- 1/2 grapefruit, peeled and segmented
- 1 cup pineapple chunks (fresh or frozen)
- 1/2 banana
- 1/2 cup Greek yogurt
- 1/2 cup orange juice
- Ice cubes (optional, for extra chill)
- Honey or maple syrup (optional, for added sweetness)

Instructions:

1. Prepare Ingredients:
   o Peel and segment the orange and grapefruit. If using fresh pineapple, cut it into chunks. Slice the banana.
2. Combine in Blender:
   o In a blender, combine the orange segments, grapefruit segments, pineapple chunks, banana slices, Greek yogurt, and orange juice.
3. Add Sweetener (Optional):
   o If you prefer a sweeter smoothie, add honey or maple syrup to the blender.
4. Include Ice Cubes (Optional):
   o For an extra refreshing and cold smoothie, add a handful of ice cubes.
5. Blend Until Smooth:
   o Blend all the ingredients until smooth and well combined. If the consistency is too thick, you can add more orange juice or water in small increments until it reaches your desired thickness.
6. Taste and Adjust:

o Taste the Citrus Sunrise Smoothie and adjust the sweetness or thickness according to your preference.

7. Pour and Serve:

   o Pour the smoothie into glasses and serve immediately.

Avocado and Spinach Detox Smoothie:

Ingredients:

- 1/2 avocado, pitted and peeled
- 1 cup fresh spinach leaves
- 1/2 cucumber, peeled and sliced
- 1/2 apple, cored and sliced
- 1/2 lemon, juiced
- 1/2 teaspoon grated ginger
- 1 cup coconut water (or water)
- Ice cubes (optional, for extra chill)
- Honey or maple syrup (optional, for added sweetness)

Instructions:

1. Prepare Ingredients:

   o Pit and peel the avocado. Wash the spinach leaves. Peel and slice the cucumber. Core and slice the apple. Juice the lemon.

2. Combine in Blender:

   o In a blender, combine the avocado, fresh spinach leaves, cucumber slices, apple slices, lemon juice, grated ginger, and coconut water.

3. Add Sweetener (Optional):

   o If you prefer a sweeter smoothie, add honey or maple syrup to the blender.

4. Include Ice Cubes (Optional):

   o For an extra refreshing and cold smoothie, add a handful of ice cubes.

5. Blend Until Smooth:

o   Blend all the ingredients until smooth and well combined. If the consistency is too thick, you can add more coconut water or water in small increments until it reaches your desired thickness.

6. Taste and Adjust:

   o   Taste the Avocado and Spinach Detox Smoothie and adjust the sweetness or thickness according to your preference.

7. Pour and Serve:

   o   Pour the smoothie into glasses and serve immediately.

Blueberry Kale Power Smoothie:

Ingredients:

- 1 cup blueberries (fresh or frozen)
- 1 cup kale leaves, stems removed
- 1/2 banana
- 1/2 cup Greek yogurt
- 1 tablespoon chia seeds
- 1 tablespoon almond butter
- 1 cup almond milk (or any milk of your choice)
- Ice cubes (optional, for extra chill)
- Honey or maple syrup (optional, for added sweetness)

Instructions:

1. Prepare Ingredients:

   o   If using fresh blueberries, wash them. Remove the stems from the kale leaves. Peel and slice the banana.

2. Combine in Blender:

   o   In a blender, combine the blueberries, kale leaves, banana slices, Greek yogurt, chia seeds, almond butter, and almond milk.

3. Add Sweetener (Optional):

   o   If you prefer a sweeter smoothie, add honey or maple syrup to the blender.

4. Include Ice Cubes (Optional):

    ○ For an extra refreshing and cold smoothie, add a handful of ice cubes.

5. Blend Until Smooth:

    ○ Blend all the ingredients until smooth and well combined. If the consistency is too thick, you can add more almond milk or water in small increments until it reaches your desired thickness.

6. Taste and Adjust:

    ○ Taste the Blueberry Kale Power Smoothie and adjust the sweetness or thickness according to your preference.

7. Pour and Serve:

    ○ Pour the smoothie into glasses and serve immediately.

Pineapple Ginger Energizing Smoothie:

Ingredients:

- 1 cup pineapple chunks (fresh or frozen)
- 1/2 banana
- 1 tablespoon fresh ginger, peeled and grated
- 1/2 cup Greek yogurt
- 1 tablespoon chia seeds
- 1 cup coconut water (or water)
- Ice cubes (optional, for extra chill)
- Honey or maple syrup (optional, for added sweetness)

Instructions:

1. Prepare Ingredients:

    ○ If using fresh pineapple, cut it into chunks. Peel and grate the fresh ginger. Peel and slice the banana.

2. Combine in Blender:

    ○ In a blender, combine the pineapple chunks, grated ginger, banana slices, Greek yogurt, chia seeds, and coconut water.

3. Add Sweetener (Optional):
   - o If you prefer a sweeter smoothie, add honey or maple syrup to the blender.
4. Include Ice Cubes (Optional):
   - o For an extra refreshing and cold smoothie, add a handful of ice cubes.
5. Blend Until Smooth:
   - o Blend all the ingredients until smooth and well combined. If the consistency is too thick, you can add more coconut water or water in small increments until it reaches your desired thickness.
6. Taste and Adjust:
   - o Taste the Pineapple Ginger Energizing Smoothie and adjust the sweetness or thickness according to your preference.
7. Pour and Serve:
   - o Pour the smoothie into glasses and serve immediately.

Cherry Almond Recovery Smoothie:

Ingredients:

- 1 cup cherries (fresh or frozen, pitted)
- 1/2 cup plain Greek yogurt
- 1/2 banana
- 1 tablespoon almond butter
- 1 tablespoon chia seeds
- 1 cup almond milk (or any milk of your choice)
- Ice cubes (optional, for extra chill)
- Honey or maple syrup (optional, for added sweetness)

Instructions:

1. Prepare Ingredients:
   - o If using fresh cherries, pit them. Peel and slice the banana.
2. Combine in Blender:

o   In a blender, combine the cherries, Greek yogurt, banana slices, almond butter, chia seeds, and almond milk.

3. Add Sweetener (Optional):

     o   If you prefer a sweeter smoothie, add honey or maple syrup to the blender.

4. Include Ice Cubes (Optional):

     o   For an extra refreshing and cold smoothie, add a handful of ice cubes.

5. Blend Until Smooth:

     o   Blend all the ingredients until smooth and well combined. If the consistency is too thick, you can add more almond milk or water in small increments until it reaches your desired thickness.

6. Taste and Adjust:

     o   Taste the Cherry Almond Recovery Smoothie and adjust the sweetness or thickness according to your preference.

7. Pour and Serve:

     o   Pour the smoothie into glasses and serve immediately.

Cucumber Mint Hydration Smoothie:

Ingredients:

- 1 cucumber, peeled and sliced
- 1/2 cup fresh mint leaves, packed
- 1/2 lime, juiced
- 1/2 green apple, cored and sliced
- 1/2 cup Greek yogurt
- 1 cup coconut water (or water)
- Ice cubes (optional, for extra chill)
- Honey or maple syrup (optional, for added sweetness)

Instructions:

1. Prepare Ingredients:

     o   Peel and slice the cucumber. Juice the lime. Core and slice the green apple.

2. Combine in Blender:
   - In a blender, combine the cucumber slices, fresh mint leaves, lime juice, green apple slices, Greek yogurt, and coconut water.
3. Add Sweetener (Optional):
   - If you prefer a sweeter smoothie, add honey or maple syrup to the blender.
4. Include Ice Cubes (Optional):
   - For an extra refreshing and cold smoothie, add a handful of ice cubes.
5. Blend Until Smooth:
   - Blend all the ingredients until smooth and well combined. If the consistency is too thick, you can add more coconut water or water in small increments until it reaches your desired thickness.
6. Taste and Adjust:
   - Taste the Cucumber Mint Hydration Smoothie and adjust the sweetness or thickness according to your preference.
7. Pour and Serve:
   - Pour the smoothie into glasses and serve immediately.

Strawberry Kiwi Antioxidant Smoothie:

Ingredients:

- 1 cup strawberries, hulled and halved
- 2 kiwis, peeled and sliced
- 1/2 banana
- 1/2 cup Greek yogurt
- 1 tablespoon chia seeds
- 1 cup orange juice
- Ice cubes (optional, for extra chill)
- Honey or maple syrup (optional, for added sweetness)

Instructions:

1. Prepare Ingredients:

o Hull and halve the strawberries. Peel and slice the kiwis. Peel and slice the banana.

2. Combine in Blender:
   o In a blender, combine the strawberries, kiwi slices, banana slices, Greek yogurt, chia seeds, and orange juice.
3. Add Sweetener (Optional):
   o If you prefer a sweeter smoothie, add honey or maple syrup to the blender.
4. Include Ice Cubes (Optional):
   o For an extra refreshing and cold smoothie, add a handful of ice cubes.
5. Blend Until Smooth:
   o Blend all the ingredients until smooth and well combined. If the consistency is too thick, you can add more orange juice or water in small increments until it reaches your desired thickness.
6. Taste and Adjust:
   o Taste the Strawberry Kiwi Antioxidant Smoothie and adjust the sweetness or thickness according to your preference.
7. Pour and Serve:
   o Pour the smoothie into glasses and serve immediately.

Papaya Coconut Paradise Smoothie:

Ingredients:

- 1 cup ripe papaya, peeled, seeded, and cubed
- 1/2 cup coconut milk
- 1/2 banana
- 1/2 cup Greek yogurt
- 1 tablespoon shredded coconut (unsweetened)
- 1 tablespoon chia seeds
- 1/2 lime, juiced
- Ice cubes (optional, for extra chill)

- Honey or maple syrup (optional, for added sweetness)

Instructions:

1. Prepare Ingredients:
   - Peel, seed, and cube the ripe papaya. Peel and slice the banana.
2. Combine in Blender:
   - In a blender, combine the papaya cubes, coconut milk, banana slices, Greek yogurt, shredded coconut, chia seeds, and lime juice.
3. Add Sweetener (Optional):
   - If you prefer a sweeter smoothie, add honey or maple syrup to the blender.
4. Include Ice Cubes (Optional):
   - For an extra refreshing and cold smoothie, add a handful of ice cubes.
5. Blend Until Smooth:
   - Blend all the ingredients until smooth and well combined. If the consistency is too thick, you can add more coconut milk or water in small increments until it reaches your desired thickness.
6. Taste and Adjust:
   - Taste the Papaya Coconut Paradise Smoothie and adjust the sweetness or thickness according to your preference.
7. Pour and Serve:
   - Pour the smoothie into glasses and serve immediately.

Chocolate Avocado Bliss Smoothie:

Ingredients:

- 1 ripe avocado, pitted and peeled
- 1 banana
- 2 tablespoons unsweetened cocoa powder
- 1 cup almond milk (or any milk of your choice)
- 1-2 tablespoons honey or maple syrup (adjust to taste)
- 1/2 teaspoon vanilla extract

- Ice cubes (optional, for extra chill)

Instructions:

1. Prepare Ingredients:
   - Pit and peel the ripe avocado. Peel the banana.
2. Combine in Blender:
   - In a blender, combine the ripe avocado, banana, unsweetened cocoa powder, almond milk, honey or maple syrup, and vanilla extract.
3. Include Ice Cubes (Optional):
   - For an extra refreshing and cold smoothie, add a handful of ice cubes.
4. Blend Until Smooth:
   - Blend all the ingredients until smooth and well combined. If the consistency is too thick, you can add more almond milk or water in small increments until it reaches your desired thickness.
5. Taste and Adjust:
   - Taste the Chocolate Avocado Bliss Smoothie and adjust the sweetness or thickness according to your preference.
6. Pour and Serve:
   - Pour the smoothie into glasses and serve immediately.

BEVERAGES:

Green Tea:

Ingredients:

- 1 teaspoon green tea leaves (or 1 green tea bag)
- 1 cup water (about 8 ounces)
- Optional: Lemon wedges, honey, or mint leaves for flavor (adjust to taste)

Instructions:

1. Boil Water:
   - Bring 1 cup of water to a boil in a kettle or saucepan.

2. Warm the Teapot or Teacup (Optional):

    o   Pour a small amount of hot water into the teapot or teacup to warm it. Swirl the water around and discard.

3. Add Green Tea Leaves or Tea Bag:

    o   Place 1 teaspoon of green tea leaves into a teapot or teacup. Alternatively, use a green tea bag.

4. Pour Hot Water:

    o   Pour the hot water over the green tea leaves or tea bag.

5. Steep the Tea:

    o   Let the green tea steep for 2-3 minutes. If you prefer a stronger flavor, you can steep for up to 5 minutes, but avoid over-steeping to prevent bitterness.

6. Strain or Remove Tea Bag:

    o   If using loose tea leaves, strain the tea to remove them. If using a tea bag, simply remove the bag.

7. Optional Additions:

    o   Customize your green tea by adding lemon wedges, a drizzle of honey or a few mint leaves for added flavor. Adjust according to your preference.

8. Serve:

    o   Pour the green tea into your favorite cup and enjoy it hot.

Turmeric Golden Milk:

Ingredients:

- 1 cup milk (dairy or plant-based, such as almond, coconut, or soy)
- 1/2 teaspoon ground turmeric
- 1/4 teaspoon ground cinnamon
- 1/4 teaspoon ground ginger
- 1 pinch black pepper (enhances turmeric absorption)
- 1 teaspoon honey or maple syrup (adjust to taste)
- 1/2 teaspoon coconut oil (optional for added richness)

Instructions:

1. Combine Ingredients:
   - In a small saucepan, combine the milk, ground turmeric, ground cinnamon, ground ginger, and a pinch of black pepper.
2. Whisk Together:
   - Whisk the ingredients together until well combined.
3. Heat Over Medium Heat:
   - Place the saucepan over medium heat and warm the mixture. Avoid boiling; a gentle simmer is sufficient.
4. Add Sweetener:
   - Stir in honey or maple syrup to sweeten the golden milk. Adjust the sweetness to your liking.
5. Optional: Add Coconut Oil for Richness:
   - For added richness and a silky texture, you can add 1/2 teaspoon of coconut oil. Stir until it melts into the golden milk.
6. Heat Through:
   - Continue to heat the golden milk until it is warmed through. Be careful not to boil.
7. Strain (Optional):
   - If you prefer a smoother texture, you can strain the golden milk to remove any sediment.
8. Pour and Serve:
   - Pour the turmeric golden milk into a cup or mug.

Cucumber Mint Infused Water:

Ingredients:

- 1/2 cucumber, thinly sliced
- 8-10 fresh mint leaves
- 1-2 liters of water (filtered or still water)

- Ice cubes (optional, for serving)

Instructions:

1. Prepare Ingredients:
   - Wash the cucumber thoroughly and slice it thinly. Rinse the mint leaves.
2. Combine in a Pitcher:
   - In a large pitcher, combine the cucumber slices and mint leaves.
3. Add Water:
   - Pour 1-2 liters of water into the pitcher, covering the cucumber and mint.
4. Refrigerate:
   - Place the pitcher in the refrigerator to chill. Allow the flavors to infuse for at least 1-2 hours, or preferably overnight for a more intense taste.
5. Serve Over Ice (Optional):
   - When ready to serve, you can add ice cubes to individual glasses for a refreshing, cold experience.

Hibiscus Tea:

Ingredients:

- 2 cups dried hibiscus petals
- 4 cups water
- 1-2 tablespoons honey or agave syrup (optional, for sweetness)
- 1 lemon or orange, sliced (optional, for citrusy flavor)
- Ice cubes (optional, for serving)

Instructions:

1. Rinse Hibiscus Petals:
   - If the dried hibiscus petals are not pre-rinsed, give them a quick rinse under cold water.
2. Boil Water:
   - In a pot, bring 4 cups of water to a boil.
3. Add Hibiscus Petals:

- Once the water is boiling, add the dried hibiscus petals to the pot. Remove the pot from heat.

4. Steep Hibiscus Tea:
   - Let the hibiscus petals steep in the hot water for about 10-15 minutes. This allows the flavors to infuse into the water.

5. Strain the Tea:
   - After steeping, strain the tea to remove the hibiscus petals. You can use a fine-mesh strainer or a piece of cheesecloth.

6. Sweeten (Optional):
   - Add honey or agave syrup to the hibiscus tea for sweetness. Adjust the amount according to your taste preferences.

7. Add Citrus (Optional):
   - For a citrusy twist, add slices of lemon or orange to the tea. This enhances the flavor and adds freshness.

8. Chill (Optional):
   - Allow the hibiscus tea to cool to room temperature. You can then refrigerate it for a few hours or serve it over ice for a refreshing iced tea.

9. Serve:
   - Pour the hibiscus tea into cups or glasses. If desired, add ice cubes for a cool experience.

Coconut Water:

Ingredients:

- 1 fresh coconut

Instructions:

1. Select a Fresh Coconut:
   - Choose a fresh coconut that feels heavy for its size and has no visible cracks.

2. Prepare the Coconut:

o Using a sturdy knife, carefully pierce one of the "eyes" or soft spots on the top of the coconut. Drain the coconut water into a bowl or glass.

3. Crack Open the Coconut:
   o To crack open the coconut, you can place it on a towel on a hard surface. Hit the coconut along its equator with the back of a heavy knife or a hammer. Rotate and repeat until it cracks open.

4. Collect Coconut Water:
   o Collect the coconut water from the cracked coconut. You can use a spoon or a coconut water extractor to scoop out the water.

5. Strain (Optional):
   o If you prefer, you can strain the coconut water through a fine-mesh sieve or cheesecloth to remove any coconut bits.

6. Chill (Optional):
   o If you like your coconut water chilled, refrigerate it for a few hours or add ice cubes before serving.

7. Serve:
   o Pour the fresh coconut water into glasses and serve immediately.

Freshly Squeezed Orange Juice:

Ingredients:

- 4-6 medium-sized oranges

Instructions:

1. Select Ripe Oranges:
   o Choose ripe and juicy oranges for the best flavor. They should feel heavy for their size and have vibrant orange skin.

2. Wash Oranges:
   o Wash the oranges thoroughly under running water to remove any dirt or residues from the skin.

3. Cut and Squeeze Oranges:

- Cut each orange in half. Using a citrus juicer, reamer, or your hands, squeeze the juice from each orange half into a bowl or a jug. Apply gentle pressure to extract the juice without incorporating too much of the bitter pith.

4. Strain (Optional):

   - If you prefer pulp-free orange juice, strain the freshly squeezed juice through a fine-mesh sieve or cheesecloth to remove any pulp.

5. Chill (Optional):

   - Refrigerate the orange juice for a few hours or serve it over ice if you prefer a chilled beverage.

6. Serve:

   - Pour the freshly squeezed orange juice into glasses.

Berry and Basil Infused Water:

Ingredients:

- 1 cup mixed berries (strawberries, blueberries, raspberries, or blackberries)
- 5-6 fresh basil leaves
- 1 liter water
- Ice cubes (optional)

Instructions:

1. Prepare Berries:

   - Wash the mixed berries thoroughly. If using strawberries, hull and slice them.

2. Crush Basil Leaves:

   - Gently crush the fresh basil leaves to release their flavor. You can use your hands or a muddler for this step.

3. Combine Ingredients:

   - In a large pitcher, combine the mixed berries and crushed basil leaves.

4. Add Water:

o   Pour 1 liter of water over the berries and basil in the pitcher.

5. Infuse:

    o   Allow the berries and basil to infuse into the water. For optimal flavor, let it sit in the refrigerator for at least 2-4 hours or overnight.

6. Serve Over Ice (Optional):

    o   If desired, serve the infused water over ice for a chilled experience.

Lemon Ginger Detox Water:

Ingredients:

- 1 lemon, thinly sliced
- 1-2 inches fresh ginger, peeled and sliced
- 1-2 tablespoons fresh mint leaves
- 1 liter water
- Ice cubes (optional)

Instructions:

1. Prepare Ingredients:

    o   Wash the lemon thoroughly and cut it into thin slices. Peel and slice the fresh ginger into thin rounds.

2. Combine Ingredients:

    o   In a large pitcher, combine the lemon slices, ginger slices, and fresh mint leaves.

3. Add Water:

    o   Pour 1 liter of water over the lemon, ginger, and mint in the pitcher.

4. Infuse:

    o   Allow the ingredients to infuse into the water. For optimal flavor, let it sit in the refrigerator for at least 2-4 hours or overnight.

5. Serve Over Ice (Optional):

    o   If desired, serve the Lemon Ginger Detox Water over ice for a refreshing and chilled experience.

Matcha Green Tea Latte:

Ingredients:

- 1 teaspoon matcha powder
- 1 tablespoon hot water (not boiling)
- 1 cup milk (dairy or plant-based)
- 1-2 teaspoons honey or sweetener of choice (optional)
- Optional: Whipped cream or frothed milk for topping

Instructions:

1. Sift Matcha Powder:
   - Sift the matcha powder into a bowl to ensure there are no lumps.
2. Whisk Matcha and Water:
   - Add the hot water to the matcha powder in the bowl. Use a bamboo matcha whisk or a small whisk to vigorously whisk the matcha and water together, creating a smooth and frothy mixture.
3. Heat Milk:
   - In a separate saucepan, heat the milk over medium heat until it's warm but not boiling.
4. Sweeten (Optional):
   - If you prefer a sweetened matcha latte, add honey or your sweetener of choice to the warmed milk. Stir until the sweetener is dissolved.
5. Combine Matcha and Milk:
   - Pour the whisked matcha into a cup. Slowly pour the warm milk over the matcha, holding back the foam with a spoon to create a layered effect.
6. Froth (Optional):
   - If desired, top the matcha latte with whipped cream or frothed milk for an extra creamy texture.

Pomegranate Juice:

Ingredients:

- 2-3 large pomegranates

Instructions:

1. Select Ripe Pomegranates:
   - Choose pomegranates that are heavy for their size and have vibrant, unblemished skin.
2. Cut Pomegranates:
   - Cut off the crown of each pomegranate, about half an inch below the crown. Score the skin in quarters from the top to the bottom.
3. Open Pomegranate:
   - Hold the pomegranate over a bowl of water, cut side down, and tap the back with a wooden spoon to release the seeds (also known as arils). The seeds will fall into the water, preventing splattering.
4. Extract Seeds:
   - Continue tapping until all the seeds are released. Alternatively, you can gently pull apart the scored sections to expose the seeds.
5. Collect Seeds:
   - Collect the seeds from the water, discarding any pith that may have fallen.
6. Blend Seeds:
   - Place the pomegranate seeds in a blender or food processor. Pulse a few times to break the seeds open without crushing them.
7. Strain Pulp:
   - Strain the blended pomegranate seeds through a fine-mesh sieve or cheesecloth into a bowl, extracting the juice. You may need to press the mixture to get all the juice.
8. Chill (Optional):
   - Refrigerate the freshly extracted pomegranate juice for a few hours if you prefer it cold.

9. Serve:

- o Pour the pomegranate juice into glasses.

Lemon Balm Tea:

Ingredients:

- 1 tablespoon fresh lemon balm leaves (or 1 teaspoon dried leaves)
- 1 cup boiling water
- Optional: Honey or sweetener of choice
- Optional: Lemon slices for garnish

Instructions:

1. Harvest or Measure Lemon Balm:
   - o If using fresh lemon balm, measure one tablespoon of leaves. If using dried lemon balm, use one teaspoon.
2. Boil Water:
   - o Bring one cup of water to a boil. You can use a kettle or a saucepan for this.
3. Prepare Lemon Balm:
   - o Place the fresh or dried lemon balm leaves in a teapot or heatproof container.
4. Pour Boiling Water:
   - o Pour the boiling water over the lemon balm leaves.
5. Steep Lemon Balm Tea:
   - o Allow the lemon balm to steep in the hot water for about 5-10 minutes. Steeping time can be adjusted based on your preference for a milder or stronger flavor.
6. Strain (Optional):
   - o If you used fresh leaves and want to remove them, strain the tea into a cup using a fine-mesh sieve or a tea strainer. If you used a tea infuser, simply remove the infuser.
7. Sweeten (Optional):

o   Add honey or your sweetener of choice to the tea, stirring until dissolved. Adjust sweetness to your liking.

8. Garnish (Optional):

   o   Garnish with a slice of lemon if desired.

9. Serve:

   o   Pour the lemon balm tea into a cup.

Almond Milk:

Ingredients:

- 1 cup raw almonds
- 4 cups water (for soaking)
- 4 cups water (for blending)
- Sweetener to taste (optional): Honey, agave syrup, or dates
- Vanilla extract (optional)

Instructions:

1. Soak Almonds:

   o   Place the almonds in a bowl and cover them with about 4 cups of water. Allow them to soak overnight or for at least 12 hours. This softens the almonds and makes them easier to blend.

2. Drain and Rinse:

   o   After soaking, drain and rinse the almonds thoroughly.

3. Blend Almonds with Water:

   o   In a blender, combine the soaked almonds and 4 cups of water. Blend on high speed until you have a smooth and creamy mixture.

4. Strain Almond Milk:

   o   Place a nut milk bag, cheesecloth, or a thin dish towel over a bowl or jug. Pour the blended almond mixture through the strainer to separate the liquid from the almond pulp.

5. Extract Liquid:

- Squeeze or press the mixture in the strainer to extract as much liquid as possible. The result is your almond milk.

6. Sweeten and Flavor (Optional):

- Add sweetener to taste, such as honey, agave syrup, or dates. If desired, add a splash of vanilla extract for flavor.

7. Store:

- Pour the almond milk into a sealable container or bottle. Store it in the refrigerator. Shake well before each use, as it may naturally separate over time.

8. Use:

- Use your homemade almond milk in coffee, tea, cereals, or as a dairy milk substitute in various recipes.

Chia Seed Lemonade:

Ingredients:

- 1/4 cup chia seeds
- 4 cups water
- 1/2 cup freshly squeezed lemon juice (about 4-5 lemons)
- 1/4 cup honey or maple syrup (adjust to taste)
- Ice cubes
- Lemon slices and mint for garnish (optional)

Instructions:

1. Prepare Chia Seeds:

- In a bowl, combine the chia seeds with 1 cup of water. Stir well to prevent clumping. Let the chia seeds sit for about 15-20 minutes, stirring occasionally. This allows the chia seeds to absorb the water and form a gel-like consistency.

2. Mix Lemon Juice and Sweetener:

- In a pitcher, combine the freshly squeezed lemon juice and honey or maple syrup. Stir until the sweetener is dissolved.

3. Add Chia Gel to Lemon Mixture:
    - Pour the chia gel into the pitcher with the lemon mixture. Stir well to combine.

4. Add Remaining Water:
    - Pour the remaining 3 cups of water into the pitcher and mix thoroughly.

5. Chill:
    - Refrigerate the Chia Seed Lemonade for at least 1-2 hours to allow the flavors to meld and the chia seeds to fully hydrate.

6. Stir Before Serving:
    - Before serving, stir the lemonade to ensure an even distribution of chia seeds.

7. Serve Over Ice:
    - Pour the Chia Seed Lemonade over ice cubes in glasses.

CHAPTER 9: SOUPS AND STEW

Spinach and Lentil Soup:

Ingredients:

- 1 cup dried green or brown lentils, rinsed and drained
- 1 tablespoon olive oil
- 1 onion, finely chopped
- 2 carrots, diced
- 2 celery stalks, diced
- 3 garlic cloves, minced
- 1 teaspoon ground cumin
- 1 teaspoon ground coriander
- 1/2 teaspoon smoked paprika
- 6 cups vegetable or chicken broth
- 1 can (14 oz) diced tomatoes
- 1 bay leaf
- Salt and pepper to taste
- 4 cups fresh spinach, chopped
- Juice of 1 lemon
- Fresh parsley for garnish (optional)

Instructions:

1. Prepare Lentils:
   - Rinse the lentils under cold water and set them aside.
2. Sauté Aromatics:
   - In a large pot, heat the olive oil over medium heat. Add chopped onion, carrots, and celery. Sauté until vegetables are softened, about 5-7 minutes.
3. Add Garlic and Spices:
   - Add minced garlic, ground cumin, ground coriander, and smoked paprika. Sauté for an additional 1-2 minutes until fragrant.

4. Combine Lentils, Broth, and Tomatoes:
   o Add the rinsed lentils to the pot, followed by the vegetable or chicken broth, diced tomatoes (with their juice), and bay leaf. Stir well.
5. Simmer:
   o Bring the soup to a boil, then reduce the heat to low, cover, and let it simmer for about 25-30 minutes or until the lentils are tender.
6. Season and Add Spinach:
   o Season the soup with salt and pepper to taste. Stir in the chopped fresh spinach and let it wilt into the soup.
7. Finish with Lemon Juice:
   o Squeeze the juice of one lemon into the soup, stirring to incorporate. Adjust the lemon juice, salt, and pepper to your taste preference.
8. Serve:
   o Ladle the Spinach and Lentil Soup into bowls. Garnish with fresh parsley if desired.

Roasted Butternut Squash Soup:

Ingredients:

- 1 large butternut squash, peeled, seeded, and diced
- 2 tablespoons olive oil
- 1 onion, chopped
- 2 carrots, chopped
- 2 celery stalks, chopped
- 3 cloves garlic, minced
- 4 cups vegetable or chicken broth
- 1 teaspoon ground cumin
- 1/2 teaspoon ground coriander
- 1/2 teaspoon smoked paprika
- Salt and pepper to taste

- 1/2 cup coconut milk or heavy cream (optional)
- Fresh thyme or parsley for garnish (optional)

Instructions:

1. Preheat Oven:
   - Preheat the oven to 400°F (200°C).
2. Roast Butternut Squash:
   - Place the diced butternut squash on a baking sheet. Drizzle with 1 tablespoon of olive oil, season with salt and pepper, and toss to coat. Roast in the preheated oven for about 25-30 minutes or until the squash is tender and lightly browned.
3. Sauté Aromatics:
   - In a large pot, heat the remaining tablespoon of olive oil over medium heat. Add chopped onion, carrots, and celery. Sauté until the vegetables are softened, about 5-7 minutes.
4. Add Garlic and Spices:
   - Add minced garlic, ground cumin, ground coriander, and smoked paprika. Sauté for an additional 1-2 minutes until fragrant.
5. Combine Roasted Squash and Broth:
   - Add the roasted butternut squash to the pot, followed by vegetable or chicken broth. Stir well to combine.
6. Simmer:
   - Bring the soup to a boil, then reduce the heat to low, cover, and let it simmer for about 15-20 minutes to allow the flavors to meld.
7. Blend Soup:
   - Use an immersion blender to puree the soup until smooth. Alternatively, transfer the soup to a blender in batches, blending until smooth. Exercise caution when blending hot liquids.
8. Season and Add Cream (Optional):

o Season the soup with salt and pepper to taste. If desired, stir in coconut milk or heavy cream for added richness.

9. Serve:

   o Ladle the Roasted Butternut Squash Soup into bowls.

Tomato Basil Soup:

Ingredients:

- 2 tablespoons olive oil
- 1 onion, chopped
- 2 carrots, chopped
- 2 celery stalks, chopped
- 3 cloves garlic, minced
- 2 cans (28 oz each) whole peeled tomatoes
- 4 cups vegetable or chicken broth
- 1 teaspoon sugar
- Salt and pepper to taste
- 1/2 cup fresh basil leaves, chopped
- 1/2 cup heavy cream (optional)
- Grated Parmesan cheese for garnish (optional)
- Croutons for serving (optional)

Instructions:

1. Sauté Aromatics:

   o In a large pot, heat the olive oil over medium heat. Add chopped onion, carrots, and celery. Sauté until the vegetables are softened, about 5-7 minutes.

2. Add Garlic and Tomatoes:

   o Add minced garlic and sauté for an additional 1-2 minutes. Add the canned tomatoes (with their juice) to the pot, breaking them up with a spoon.

3. Simmer:

- o Pour in the vegetable or chicken broth. Add sugar, salt, and pepper to taste. Bring the soup to a boil, then reduce the heat to low, cover, and let it simmer for about 15-20 minutes.

4. Blend Soup:
   - o Use an immersion blender to puree the soup until smooth. Alternatively, transfer the soup to a blender in batches, blending until smooth. Exercise caution when blending hot liquids.

5. Add Basil:
   - o Stir in the chopped fresh basil and let the soup simmer for an additional 5 minutes.

6. Add Cream (Optional):
   - o If desired, stir in heavy cream for added richness. Adjust the seasoning as needed.

7. Serve:
   - o Ladle the Tomato Basil Soup into bowls.

Mushroom Barley Soup:

Ingredients:

- 1 cup pearl barley
- 2 tablespoons olive oil
- 1 onion, finely chopped
- 2 carrots, diced
- 2 celery stalks, diced
- 3 cloves garlic, minced
- 8 oz (about 227g) cremini or button mushrooms, sliced
- 6 cups vegetable or beef broth
- 1 teaspoon dried thyme
- 1 bay leaf
- Salt and pepper to taste

- 1/4 cup soy sauce (optional, for extra depth of flavor)
- Fresh parsley for garnish (optional)

Instructions:

1. Rinse Barley:
   - Rinse the pearl barley under cold water and set it aside.
2. Sauté Vegetables:
   - In a large pot, heat the olive oil over medium heat. Add chopped onion, carrots, and celery. Sauté until the vegetables are softened, about 5-7 minutes.
3. Add Garlic and Mushrooms:
   - Add minced garlic and sliced mushrooms to the pot. Sauté for an additional 3-5 minutes until the mushrooms release their moisture.
4. Add Barley and Broth:
   - Add the rinsed barley to the pot, followed by vegetable or beef broth. Stir well.
5. Season and Simmer:
   - Add dried thyme, bay leaf, salt, and pepper to taste. If using, stir in soy sauce for extra depth of flavor. Bring the soup to a boil, then reduce the heat to low, cover, and let it simmer for about 40-50 minutes or until the barley is tender.
6. Adjust Seasoning:
   - Taste the soup and adjust the seasoning if necessary. Remove the bay leaf.
7. Serve:
   - Ladle the Mushroom Barley Soup into bowls.

Chicken and Vegetable Broth:

Ingredients:

- 1 whole chicken (about 3-4 pounds), cleaned and giblets removed
- 8 cups water

- 2 carrots, chopped
- 2 celery stalks, chopped
- 1 onion, quartered
- 3 cloves garlic, smashed
- 1 parsnip, chopped (optional)
- 1 leek, cleaned and sliced (optional)
- 2 bay leaves
- 1 teaspoon whole peppercorns
- Salt to taste
- Fresh parsley for garnish (optional)

Instructions:

1. Prepare Chicken:
   - Rinse the whole chicken under cold water and pat it dry with paper towels.
2. Boil Chicken:
   - In a large stockpot, combine the whole chicken and 8 cups of water. Bring to a boil over medium-high heat. Skim off any foam or impurities that rise to the surface.
3. Add Vegetables:
   - Add chopped carrots, celery, onion, garlic, parsnip (if using), leek (if using), bay leaves, and peppercorns to the pot.
4. Simmer:
   - Reduce the heat to low, cover the pot, and let the broth simmer gently for about 1.5 to 2 hours. This allows the flavors to meld and the chicken to become tender.
5. Season:
   - Season the broth with salt to taste. Adjust the seasoning as needed.
6. Strain:

o Carefully remove the chicken from the pot. Strain the broth through a fine-mesh sieve or cheesecloth into another large pot or bowl. Discard the solids (vegetables and chicken bones).

7. Shred Chicken (Optional):

   o If you want to use the cooked chicken meat, let it cool slightly, then shred the meat from the bones. Add the shredded chicken back into the strained broth if desired.

8. Serve:

   o Ladle the Chicken and Vegetable Broth into bowls.

Turmeric Carrot Ginger Soup:

Ingredients:

- 1 tablespoon olive oil
- 1 onion, chopped
- 1 pound carrots, peeled and chopped
- 2 tablespoons fresh ginger, grated
- 3 cloves garlic, minced
- 1 teaspoon ground turmeric
- 1/2 teaspoon ground cumin
- 6 cups vegetable or chicken broth
- Salt and pepper to taste
- 1 can (14 oz) coconut milk
- Juice of 1 lemon
- Fresh cilantro for garnish (optional)

Instructions:

1. Sauté Aromatics:

   o In a large pot, heat the olive oil over medium heat. Add chopped onion, carrots, and grated ginger. Sauté until the vegetables are softened, about 5-7 minutes.

2. Add Garlic and Spices:

   - Add minced garlic, ground turmeric, and ground cumin. Sauté for an additional 1-2 minutes until fragrant.

3. Add Broth:

   - Pour in the vegetable or chicken broth, scraping any bits from the bottom of the pot. Bring the soup to a boil.

4. Simmer:

   - Reduce the heat to low, cover the pot, and let it simmer for about 15-20 minutes or until the carrots are tender.

5. Blend Soup:

   - Use an immersion blender to puree the soup until smooth. Alternatively, transfer the soup to a blender in batches, blending until smooth. Exercise caution when blending hot liquids.

6. Season:

   - Season the soup with salt and pepper to taste.

7. Add Coconut Milk and Lemon Juice:

   - Stir in the coconut milk and lemon juice. Heat the soup for an additional 5 minutes, allowing the flavors to meld.

8. Adjust Consistency (Optional):

   - If the soup is too thick, you can add more broth or coconut milk to reach your desired consistency.

9. Serve:

   - Ladle the Turmeric Carrot Ginger Soup into bowls.

Kale and White Bean Soup:

Ingredients:

- 1 tablespoon olive oil
- 1 onion, chopped
- 2 carrots, diced

- 2 celery stalks, diced
- 3 cloves garlic, minced
- 1 teaspoon dried thyme
- 1 teaspoon dried rosemary
- 1 can (14 oz) white beans (cannellini or navy), drained and rinsed
- 4 cups vegetable or chicken broth
- 1 bunch kale, stems removed and leaves chopped
- Salt and pepper to taste
- Juice of 1 lemon
- Grated Parmesan cheese for garnish (optional)

Instructions:

1. Sauté Aromatics:
   - In a large pot, heat the olive oil over medium heat. Add chopped onion, diced carrots, and diced celery. Sauté until the vegetables are softened, about 5-7 minutes.
2. Add Garlic and Herbs:
   - Add minced garlic, dried thyme, and dried rosemary. Sauté for an additional 1-2 minutes until fragrant.
3. Add White Beans and Broth:
   - Add the drained and rinsed white beans to the pot. Pour in the vegetable or chicken broth. Stir well.
4. Simmer:
   - Bring the soup to a boil, then reduce the heat to low, cover, and let it simmer for about 15-20 minutes to allow the flavors to meld.
5. Add Kale:
   - Add the chopped kale to the pot. Stir and let the kale wilt into the soup. Simmer for an additional 5-7 minutes until the kale is tender.
6. Season:
   - Season the soup with salt and pepper to taste.

7. Add Lemon Juice:

    o Squeeze the juice of one lemon into the soup, stirring to incorporate. Adjust the lemon juice, salt, and pepper to your taste.

8. Serve:

    o Ladle the Kale and White Bean Soup into bowls.

Chicken and Rice Soup:

Ingredients:

- 1 tablespoon olive oil
- 1 onion, chopped
- 2 carrots, diced
- 2 celery stalks, diced
- 3 cloves garlic, minced
- 1 teaspoon dried thyme
- 1 teaspoon dried rosemary
- 1 cup uncooked white rice
- 6 cups chicken broth
- 1 pound boneless, skinless chicken breasts or thighs, cooked and shredded
- Salt and pepper to taste
- Fresh parsley for garnish (optional)
- Lemon wedges for serving (optional)

Instructions:

1. Sauté Aromatics:

    o In a large pot, heat the olive oil over medium heat. Add chopped onion, diced carrots, and diced celery. Sauté until the vegetables are softened, about 5-7 minutes.

2. Add Garlic and Herbs:

    o Add minced garlic, dried thyme, and dried rosemary. Sauté for an additional 1-2 minutes until fragrant.

3. Add Rice and Broth:

   o Add the uncooked rice to the pot. Pour in the chicken broth. Stir well.

4. Simmer Rice:

   o Bring the soup to a boil, then reduce the heat to low, cover, and let it simmer for about 15-20 minutes or until the rice is cooked.

5. Add Shredded Chicken:

   o Stir in the cooked and shredded chicken. Let the soup simmer for an additional 5-7 minutes to allow the flavors to meld.

6. Season:

   o Season the soup with salt and pepper to taste.

7. Serve:

   o Ladle the Chicken and Rice Soup into bowls.

Quinoa Minestrone Soup:

Ingredients:

- 1 tablespoon olive oil
- 1 onion, chopped
- 2 carrots, diced
- 2 celery stalks, diced
- 3 cloves garlic, minced
- 1 teaspoon dried oregano
- 1 teaspoon dried basil
- 1 can (14 oz) diced tomatoes
- 1/2 cup quinoa, rinsed and drained
- 6 cups vegetable broth
- 1 can (15 oz) kidney beans, drained and rinsed
- 1 zucchini, diced
- 1 cup green beans, chopped
- 1 cup chopped kale or spinach

- Salt and pepper to taste
- Grated Parmesan cheese for serving (optional)
- Fresh basil for garnish (optional)

Instructions:

1. Sauté Aromatics:
   - In a large pot, heat the olive oil over medium heat. Add chopped onion, diced carrots, and diced celery. Sauté until the vegetables are softened, about 5-7 minutes.
2. Add Garlic and Herbs:
   - Add minced garlic, dried oregano, and dried basil. Sauté for an additional 1-2 minutes until fragrant.
3. Add Tomatoes and Quinoa:
   - Add the diced tomatoes (with their juice) to the pot. Stir in the rinsed quinoa.
4. Pour in Broth:
   - Pour in the vegetable broth. Stir well.
5. Simmer Quinoa:
   - Bring the soup to a boil, then reduce the heat to low, cover, and let it simmer for about 15 minutes.
6. Add Beans and Vegetables:
   - Stir in the drained and rinsed kidney beans, diced zucchini, chopped green beans, and chopped kale or spinach.
7. Continue Simmering:
   - Continue simmering the soup for an additional 15-20 minutes or until the quinoa and vegetables are tender.
8. Season:
   - Season the Minestrone Soup with salt and pepper to taste.
9. Serve:
   - Ladle the Quinoa Minestrone Soup into bowls.

Sweet Potato and Black Bean Soup:

Ingredients:

- 1 tablespoon olive oil
- 1 onion, chopped
- 2 cloves garlic, minced
- 1 teaspoon ground cumin
- 1 teaspoon ground coriander
- 1/2 teaspoon smoked paprika
- 2 large sweet potatoes, peeled and diced
- 1 can (15 oz) black beans, drained and rinsed
- 1 can (14 oz) diced tomatoes
- 6 cups vegetable broth
- Salt and pepper to taste
- Juice of 1 lime
- Fresh cilantro for garnish (optional)
- Sour cream or Greek yogurt for topping (optional)
- Avocado slices for topping (optional)

Instructions:

1. Sauté Aromatics:
   - In a large pot, heat the olive oil over medium heat. Add chopped onion and sauté until softened, about 5 minutes. Add minced garlic and sauté for an additional 1-2 minutes.
2. Add Spices:
   - Stir in ground cumin, ground coriander, and smoked paprika. Sauté for another minute until the spices are fragrant.
3. Add Sweet Potatoes:
   - Add the diced sweet potatoes to the pot. Stir to coat them with the aromatic mixture.
4. Add Black Beans, Tomatoes, and Broth:

- Add black beans, diced tomatoes (with their juice), and vegetable broth to the pot. Stir well.

5. Simmer:

    - Bring the soup to a boil, then reduce the heat to low, cover, and let it simmer for about 20-25 minutes or until the sweet potatoes are tender.

6. Season:

    - Season the Sweet Potato and Black Bean Soup with salt and pepper to taste.

7. Add Lime Juice:

    - Squeeze the juice of one lime into the soup, stirring to incorporate. Adjust the lime juice, salt, and pepper to your taste.

8. Serve:

    - Ladle the soup into bowls.

Lemon Garlic Chicken Soup:

Ingredients:

- 1 tablespoon olive oil
- 1 onion, chopped
- 2 carrots, diced
- 2 celery stalks, diced
- 3 cloves garlic, minced
- 1 teaspoon dried thyme
- 1 teaspoon dried rosemary
- 6 cups chicken broth
- 1 pound boneless, skinless chicken breasts, cooked and shredded
- 1/2 cup orzo or small pasta
- Juice of 2 lemons
- Zest of 1 lemon
- Salt and pepper to taste
- Fresh parsley for garnish (optional)

Instructions:

1. Sauté Aromatics:
   - o In a large pot, heat the olive oil over medium heat. Add chopped onion, diced carrots, and diced celery. Sauté until the vegetables are softened, about 5-7 minutes.
2. Add Garlic and Herbs:
   - o Add minced garlic, dried thyme, and dried rosemary. Sauté for an additional 1-2 minutes until fragrant.
3. Pour in Broth:
   - o Pour in the chicken broth. Stir well.
4. Add Shredded Chicken:
   - o Add the cooked and shredded chicken to the pot. Bring the soup to a gentle boil.
5. Add Orzo or Pasta:
   - o Stir in the orzo or small pasta. Cook according to package instructions until al dente.
6. Lemon Infusion:
   - o Add the juice of 2 lemons and the zest of 1 lemon to the soup. Stir well to infuse the soup with lemon flavor.
7. Season:
   - o Season the Lemon Garlic Chicken Soup with salt and pepper to taste.
8. Simmer:
   - o Let the soup simmer for an additional 5-7 minutes to allow the flavors to meld.
9. Serve:
   - o Ladle the soup into bowls.

Cauliflower and Broccoli Soup:

Ingredients:

- 1 tablespoon olive oil
- 1 onion, chopped
- 2 cloves garlic, minced
- 1 head cauliflower, chopped into florets
- 1 head broccoli, chopped into florets
- 4 cups vegetable broth
- 1 teaspoon dried thyme
- 1/2 teaspoon ground nutmeg
- Salt and pepper to taste
- 1 cup unsweetened almond milk or regular milk
- 1/4 cup grated Parmesan cheese (optional)
- Fresh chives or parsley for garnish (optional)

Instructions:

1. Sauté Aromatics:
   - In a large pot, heat the olive oil over medium heat. Add chopped onion and sauté until softened, about 5 minutes. Add minced garlic and sauté for an additional 1-2 minutes.
2. Add Cauliflower and Broccoli:
   - Add the cauliflower and broccoli florets to the pot. Stir well.
3. Pour in Broth:
   - Pour in the vegetable broth. Stir in dried thyme, ground nutmeg, salt, and pepper to taste.
4. Simmer:
   - Bring the soup to a boil, then reduce the heat to low, cover, and let it simmer for about 20-25 minutes or until the cauliflower and broccoli are tender.
5. Blend Soup:

o Use an immersion blender to puree the soup until smooth. Alternatively, transfer the soup to a blender in batches, blending until smooth. Exercise caution when blending hot liquids.

6. Add Milk:

    o Stir in the almond milk or regular milk. Adjust the consistency to your liking by adding more milk if needed.

7. Season and Optional Cheese:

    o Season the Cauliflower and Broccoli Soup with additional salt and pepper if necessary. If desired, stir in grated Parmesan cheese for added richness.

8. Serve:

    o Ladle the soup into bowls.

Beet and Orange Soup:

Ingredients:

- 1 tablespoon olive oil
- 1 onion, chopped
- 3 beets, peeled and diced
- 3 carrots, peeled and diced
- 3 cups vegetable broth
- 2 oranges, juiced and zested
- 1 teaspoon ground cumin
- 1 teaspoon coriander
- Salt and pepper to taste
- Greek yogurt or sour cream for serving
- Fresh dill for garnish (optional)

Instructions:

1. Sauté Aromatics:

    o In a large pot, heat the olive oil over medium heat. Add chopped onion and sauté until softened, about 5 minutes.

2. Add Beets and Carrots:
   - Add diced beets and carrots to the pot. Stir well.
3. Pour in Broth:
   - Pour in the vegetable broth. Bring the soup to a boil, then reduce the heat to low, cover, and let it simmer for about 20-25 minutes or until the beets and carrots are tender.
4. Blend Soup:
   - Use an immersion blender to puree the soup until smooth. Alternatively, transfer the soup to a blender in batches, blending until smooth. Exercise caution when blending hot liquids.
5. Add Orange Juice and Zest:
   - Stir in the freshly squeezed orange juice and the zest of one orange. Mix well.
6. Season with Spices:
   - Add ground cumin, coriander, salt, and pepper to taste. Adjust the seasoning as needed.
7. Simmer:
   - Let the soup simmer for an additional 5 minutes to allow the flavors to meld.
8. Serve:
   - Ladle the Beet and Orange Soup into bowls.

Zucchini Noodle Chicken Soup:

Ingredients:

- 1 tablespoon olive oil
- 1 onion, chopped
- 2 carrots, diced
- 2 celery stalks, diced
- 3 cloves garlic, minced

- 1 teaspoon dried thyme
- 6 cups chicken broth
- 1 pound boneless, skinless chicken breasts, cooked and shredded
- 3 medium zucchinis, spiralized into noodles
- Salt and pepper to taste
- Juice of 1 lemon
- Fresh parsley for garnish (optional)

Instructions:

1. Sauté Aromatics:
   - o In a large pot, heat the olive oil over medium heat. Add chopped onion, diced carrots, and diced celery. Sauté until the vegetables are softened, about 5-7 minutes.
2. Add Garlic and Thyme:
   - o Add minced garlic and dried thyme. Sauté for an additional 1-2 minutes until fragrant.
3. Pour in Broth:
   - o Pour in the chicken broth. Bring the soup to a gentle boil.
4. Add Shredded Chicken:
   - o Add the cooked and shredded chicken to the pot. Stir well.
5. Simmer:
   - o Let the soup simmer for about 10-15 minutes to allow the flavors to meld.
6. Add Zucchini Noodles:
   - o Add the spiralized zucchini noodles to the pot. Cook for an additional 3-5 minutes until the zucchini noodles are tender but still have a bit of bite.
7. Season:
   - o Season the Zucchini Noodle Chicken Soup with salt and pepper to taste.
8. Add Lemon Juice:
   - o Squeeze the juice of one lemon into the soup, stirring to incorporate. Adjust the lemon juice, salt, and pepper to your taste.

9. Serve:

- Ladle the soup into bowls.

Lentil and Kale Detox Soup:

Ingredients:

- 1 tablespoon olive oil
- 1 onion, chopped
- 2 carrots, diced
- 2 celery stalks, diced
- 3 cloves garlic, minced
- 1 cup dried green or brown lentils, rinsed and drained
- 8 cups vegetable broth
- 1 teaspoon ground cumin
- 1 teaspoon ground turmeric
- 1/2 teaspoon smoked paprika
- 1 bay leaf
- Salt and pepper to taste
- 1 bunch kale, stems removed and leaves chopped
- Juice of 1 lemon
- Fresh cilantro or parsley for garnish (optional)

Instructions:

1. Sauté Aromatics:
   - In a large pot, heat the olive oil over medium heat. Add chopped onion, diced carrots, and diced celery. Sauté until the vegetables are softened, about 5-7 minutes.
2. Add Garlic and Lentils:
   - Add minced garlic and rinsed lentils to the pot. Stir well.
3. Pour in Broth:

o   Pour in the vegetable broth. Stir in ground cumin, ground turmeric, smoked paprika, bay leaf, salt, and pepper to taste.

4. Simmer Lentils:

o   Bring the soup to a boil, then reduce the heat to low, cover, and let it simmer for about 20-25 minutes or until the lentils are tender.

5. Add Kale:

o   Add the chopped kale to the pot. Stir and let the kale wilt into the soup. Simmer for an additional 5-7 minutes until the kale is tender.

6. Season and Lemon Juice:

o   Season the Lentil and Kale Detox Soup with salt and pepper to taste. Squeeze the juice of one lemon into the soup, stirring to incorporate. Adjust the lemon juice, salt, and pepper to your taste.

7. Serve:

o   Ladle the soup into bowls.

STEWS:

Vegetarian Chili:

Ingredients:

- 2 tablespoons olive oil
- 1 onion, chopped
- 3 cloves garlic, minced
- 1 bell pepper, diced (any color)
- 1 zucchini, diced
- 1 carrot, diced
- 1 jalapeño, finely chopped (optional, for heat)
- 2 cans (14 oz each) diced tomatoes
- 1 can (15 oz) black beans, drained and rinsed
- 1 can (15 oz) kidney beans, drained and rinsed

- 1 can (15 oz) corn kernels, drained
- 1 cup vegetable broth
- 2 tablespoons tomato paste
- 2 teaspoons ground cumin
- 2 teaspoons chili powder
- 1 teaspoon smoked paprika
- 1 teaspoon dried oregano
- Salt and pepper to taste
- Lime wedges for serving
- Fresh cilantro for garnish
- Shredded cheese, sour cream, or avocado for topping (optional)

Instructions:

1. Sauté Aromatics:
   - In a large pot, heat olive oil over medium heat. Add chopped onion, minced garlic, diced bell pepper, diced zucchini, diced carrot, and chopped jalapeño (if using). Sauté until vegetables are softened, about 5-7 minutes.
2. Add Tomatoes and Tomato Paste:
   - Add diced tomatoes (with their juice) and tomato paste to the pot. Stir well.
3. Add Beans, Corn, and Broth:
   - Add black beans, kidney beans, corn kernels, and vegetable broth to the pot. Stir to combine.
4. Season:
   - Stir in ground cumin, chili powder, smoked paprika, dried oregano, salt, and pepper to taste.
5. Simmer:
   - Bring the chili to a boil, then reduce the heat to low. Cover and let it simmer for about 20-30 minutes to allow the flavors to meld.
6. Adjust Consistency:

o If the chili is too thick, you can add more vegetable broth to reach your desired consistency.

7. Taste and Adjust:

    o Taste the chili and adjust the seasoning as needed.

8. Serve:

    o Ladle the Vegetarian Chili into bowls.

Moroccan Chickpea Stew:

Ingredients:

- 2 tablespoons olive oil
- 1 onion, finely chopped
- 3 cloves garlic, minced
- 1 teaspoon ground cumin
- 1 teaspoon ground coriander
- 1 teaspoon ground turmeric
- 1/2 teaspoon ground cinnamon
- 1/4 teaspoon cayenne pepper (adjust to taste)
- 1 can (14 oz) diced tomatoes
- 2 cans (15 oz each) chickpeas, drained and rinsed
- 1 sweet potato, peeled and diced
- 3 carrots, peeled and sliced
- 4 cups vegetable broth
- 1 tablespoon tomato paste
- 1 preserved lemon, flesh removed, peel thinly sliced (or substitute with 1 fresh lemon, zest and juice)
- Salt and pepper to taste
- Fresh cilantro for garnish
- Cooked couscous or rice for serving

Instructions:

1. Sauté Aromatics:
    - In a large pot, heat olive oil over medium heat. Add finely chopped onion and sauté until softened, about 5 minutes. Add minced garlic and sauté for an additional 1-2 minutes.
2. Add Spices:
    - Stir in ground cumin, ground coriander, ground turmeric, ground cinnamon, and cayenne pepper. Sauté for another minute until the spices are fragrant.
3. Add Tomatoes and Chickpeas:
    - Add diced tomatoes (with their juice) and drained chickpeas to the pot. Stir well.
4. Add Vegetables and Broth:
    - Add diced sweet potato, sliced carrots, vegetable broth, and tomato paste. Stir to combine.
5. Simmer:
    - Bring the stew to a boil, then reduce the heat to low. Cover and let it simmer for about 25-30 minutes or until the vegetables are tender.
6. Add Preserved Lemon:
    - Stir in the thinly sliced preserved lemon peel (or lemon zest and juice). Season with salt and pepper to taste.
7. Adjust Consistency:
    - If the stew is too thick, you can add more vegetable broth.
8. Serve:
    - Serve the Moroccan Chickpea Stew over cooked couscous or rice.

Turkey and Sweet Potato Stew:

Ingredients:

- 1 tablespoon olive oil
- 1 onion, chopped
- 2 cloves garlic, minced

- 1 pound ground turkey
- 2 sweet potatoes, peeled and diced
- 3 carrots, peeled and sliced
- 1 bell pepper, diced (any color)
- 1 can (14 oz) diced tomatoes
- 4 cups chicken broth
- 1 teaspoon dried thyme
- 1 teaspoon dried rosemary
- 1/2 teaspoon smoked paprika
- Salt and pepper to taste
- 1 cup frozen peas
- Fresh parsley for garnish (optional)

Instructions:

1. Sauté Aromatics:
   - In a large pot, heat olive oil over medium heat. Add chopped onion and sauté until softened, about 5 minutes. Add minced garlic and sauté for an additional 1-2 minutes.
2. Cook Turkey:
   - Add ground turkey to the pot. Cook, breaking it apart with a spoon, until browned and cooked through.
3. Add Vegetables:
   - Stir in diced sweet potatoes, sliced carrots, and diced bell pepper.
4. Pour in Broth and Tomatoes:
   - Pour in chicken broth and add diced tomatoes (with their juice). Stir well.
5. Season:
   - Stir in dried thyme, dried rosemary, smoked paprika, salt, and pepper to taste.
6. Simmer:

- Bring the stew to a boil, then reduce the heat to low. Cover and let it simmer for about 20-25 minutes or until the sweet potatoes and carrots are tender.

7. Add Peas:
   - Stir in frozen peas and let them cook for an additional 3-5 minutes.
8. Adjust Consistency and Seasoning:
   - If needed, adjust the consistency with more broth. Taste and adjust the seasoning.
9. Serve:
   - Ladle the Turkey and Sweet Potato Stew into bowls.

Beef and Vegetable Stew:

Ingredients:

- 1.5 pounds stewing beef, cut into bite-sized pieces
- 2 tablespoons olive oil
- 1 onion, chopped
- 3 cloves garlic, minced
- 2 carrots, peeled and sliced
- 2 parsnips, peeled and sliced
- 2 potatoes, peeled and diced
- 1 cup green beans, trimmed and cut into bite-sized pieces
- 1 can (14 oz) diced tomatoes
- 4 cups beef broth
- 2 tablespoons tomato paste
- 1 teaspoon dried thyme
- 1 teaspoon dried rosemary
- 1 bay leaf
- Salt and pepper to taste
- 1 cup frozen peas

- Fresh parsley for garnish (optional)

Instructions:

1. Brown Beef:
   - In a large pot, heat olive oil over medium-high heat. Add stewing beef and brown on all sides. Remove beef from the pot and set aside.
2. Sauté Aromatics:
   - In the same pot, add chopped onion and sauté until softened, about 5 minutes. Add minced garlic and sauté for an additional 1-2 minutes.
3. Add Vegetables:
   - Return the browned beef to the pot. Add sliced carrots, sliced parsnips, diced potatoes, and green beans.
4. Pour in Broth and Tomatoes:
   - Pour in beef broth and add diced tomatoes (with their juice). Stir well.
5. Add Tomato Paste and Herbs:
   - Stir in tomato paste, dried thyme, dried rosemary, bay leaf, salt, and pepper to taste.
6. Simmer:
   - Bring the stew to a boil, then reduce the heat to low. Cover and let it simmer for about 1.5 to 2 hours, or until the beef is tender.
7. Add Peas:
   - Stir in frozen peas and let them cook for an additional 5-7 minutes.
8. Adjust Consistency and Seasoning:
   - If needed, adjust the consistency with more broth. Taste and adjust the seasoning.
9. Serve:
   - Ladle the Beef and Vegetable Stew into bowls.

Coconut Curry Lentil Stew:

Ingredients:

- 1 cup dried green or brown lentils, rinsed
- 1 can (14 oz) coconut milk (light or regular)
- 1 onion, finely chopped
- 2 cloves garlic, minced
- 1 tablespoon fresh ginger, grated
- 1 sweet potato, peeled and diced
- 1 cup cherry tomatoes, halved
- 1 cup spinach or kale, chopped
- 2 tablespoons curry powder
- 1 teaspoon turmeric powder
- 1 teaspoon cumin
- 1 tablespoon coconut oil
- Salt and pepper to taste
- Fresh cilantro for garnish (optional)
- Lime wedges for serving

Instructions:

1. In a large pot, heat coconut oil over medium heat. Add chopped onions and cook until they become translucent.
2. Add minced garlic and grated ginger to the pot, stirring for about a minute until fragrant.
3. Stir in curry powder, turmeric, and cumin, allowing the spices to toast for another minute.
4. Add lentils, diced sweet potato, and coconut milk to the pot. Bring to a simmer and let it cook for about 20-25 minutes or until lentils and sweet potatoes are tender.
5. Add cherry tomatoes and chopped spinach or kale to the stew, letting them cook for an additional 5-7 minutes until the vegetables are cooked through.
6. Season the stew with salt and pepper to taste.

7. Serve the Coconut Curry Lentil Stew hot, garnished with fresh cilantro if desired, and accompanied by lime wedges for a burst of citrus flavor.

White Bean and Kale Stew:

Ingredients:

- 2 cans (15 oz each) white beans (cannellini or Great Northern), drained and rinsed
- 1 bunch of kale, stems removed and leaves chopped
- 1 onion, finely chopped
- 3 cloves garlic, minced
- 2 carrots, peeled and diced
- 2 celery stalks, diced
- 1 can (14 oz) diced tomatoes (fire-roasted for extra flavor)
- 4 cups vegetable broth
- 1 teaspoon dried thyme
- 1 teaspoon dried rosemary
- 1 bay leaf
- 2 tablespoons olive oil
- Salt and pepper to taste
- Grated Parmesan cheese for serving (optional)

Instructions:

1. In a large pot, heat olive oil over medium heat. Add chopped onion, garlic, carrots, and celery. Sauté until the vegetables are softened.
2. Add chopped kale to the pot and cook until it wilts down.
3. Pour in the vegetable broth, diced tomatoes (with their juice), drained white beans, thyme, rosemary, and bay leaf. Stir to combine.
4. Bring the stew to a simmer, then reduce the heat to low, cover, and let it simmer for about 20-25 minutes to allow the flavors to meld.
5. Season the stew with salt and pepper to taste. Adjust the seasoning as needed.
6. Remove the bay leaf and discard.

7. Serve the White Bean and Kale Stew hot, optionally topped with grated Parmesan cheese for extra flavor.

Chicken and Quinoa Stew:

Ingredients:

- 1 pound boneless, skinless chicken breasts, cut into bite-sized pieces
- 1 cup quinoa, rinsed
- 1 onion, finely chopped
- 3 carrots, peeled and diced
- 2 celery stalks, diced
- 3 cloves garlic, minced
- 1 can (14 oz) diced tomatoes
- 6 cups chicken broth
- 1 teaspoon dried thyme
- 1 teaspoon dried rosemary
- 1 bay leaf
- Salt and pepper to taste
- 2 tablespoons olive oil
- Fresh parsley for garnish (optional)

Instructions:

1. In a large pot, heat olive oil over medium heat. Add chopped onion, garlic, carrots, and celery. Sauté until the vegetables are softened.
2. Add the chicken pieces to the pot and cook until they are browned on all sides.
3. Pour in the chicken broth, diced tomatoes (with their juice), and rinsed quinoa. Stir to combine.
4. Add dried thyme, rosemary, and the bay leaf to the pot. Season with salt and pepper to taste.

5. Bring the stew to a simmer, then reduce the heat to low, cover, and let it simmer for about 20-25 minutes or until the chicken is cooked through, and the quinoa is tender.

6. Taste and adjust the seasoning if necessary. Remove the bay leaf and discard.

7. Serve the Chicken and Quinoa Stew hot, garnished with fresh parsley if desired.

Tomato and Eggplant Stew:

Ingredients:

- 1 large eggplant, diced
- 1 onion, finely chopped
- 3 cloves garlic, minced
- 1 can (14 oz) diced tomatoes
- 1 can (6 oz) tomato paste
- 1 bell pepper, diced
- 2 tablespoons olive oil
- 1 teaspoon dried oregano
- 1 teaspoon dried basil
- 1 teaspoon paprika
- Salt and pepper to taste
- Fresh basil for garnish (optional)

Instructions:

1. In a large pot, heat olive oil over medium heat. Add chopped onion and garlic. Sauté until the onions are translucent.

2. Add diced eggplant to the pot and cook until it begins to soften.

3. Stir in diced tomatoes, tomato paste, and diced bell pepper. Mix well.

4. Season the stew with dried oregano, dried basil, paprika, salt, and pepper. Stir to combine.

5. Cover the pot and let the stew simmer on low heat for about 20-25 minutes, or until the eggplant is tender and the flavors have melded.

6. Taste and adjust the seasoning if needed.

7. Serve the Tomato and Eggplant Stew hot, garnished with fresh basil if desired.

Black-Eyed Pea and Collard Green Stew:

Ingredients:

- 2 cans (15 oz each) black-eyed peas, drained and rinsed
- 1 bunch of collard greens, stems removed and leaves chopped
- 1 onion, finely chopped
- 3 cloves garlic, minced
- 2 carrots, peeled and diced
- 2 celery stalks, diced
- 1 can (14 oz) diced tomatoes
- 6 cups vegetable broth
- 1 teaspoon smoked paprika
- 1 teaspoon cumin
- 1 bay leaf
- Salt and pepper to taste
- 2 tablespoons olive oil
- Hot sauce for serving (optional)

Instructions:

1. In a large pot, heat olive oil over medium heat. Add chopped onion, garlic, carrots, and celery. Sauté until the vegetables are softened.

2. Add chopped collard greens to the pot and cook until they wilt down.

3. Pour in the vegetable broth, diced tomatoes (with their juice), and drained black-eyed peas. Stir to combine.

4. Add smoked paprika, cumin, and the bay leaf to the pot. Season with salt and pepper to taste.

5. Bring the stew to a simmer, then reduce the heat to low, cover, and let it simmer for about 20-25 minutes or until the collard greens are tender.

6. Taste and adjust the seasoning if necessary. Remove the bay leaf and discard.

7. Serve the Black-Eyed Pea and Collard Green Stew hot, with a dash of hot sauce if desired.

Spiced Lentil and Pumpkin Stew:

Ingredients:

- 1 cup dried brown or green lentils, rinsed
- 2 cups pumpkin or butternut squash, peeled and diced
- 1 onion, finely chopped
- 3 cloves garlic, minced
- 1 can (14 oz) diced tomatoes
- 4 cups vegetable broth
- 2 tablespoons tomato paste
- 1 teaspoon ground cumin
- 1 teaspoon ground coriander
- 1/2 teaspoon ground turmeric
- 1/2 teaspoon smoked paprika
- 1/4 teaspoon cayenne pepper (adjust to taste)
- Salt and pepper to taste
- 2 tablespoons olive oil
- Fresh cilantro for garnish (optional)

Instructions:

1. In a large pot, heat olive oil over medium heat. Add chopped onion and garlic. Sauté until the onions are translucent.

2. Add diced pumpkin or butternut squash to the pot and cook for a few minutes until they start to soften.

3. Pour in the vegetable broth, diced tomatoes (with their juice), and rinsed lentils. Stir to combine.

4. Add tomato paste, ground cumin, ground coriander, ground turmeric, smoked paprika, cayenne pepper, salt, and pepper to the pot. Mix well.

5. Bring the stew to a simmer, then reduce the heat to low, cover, and let it simmer for about 20-25 minutes or until the lentils are tender and the pumpkin is cooked through.

6. Taste and adjust the seasoning if necessary.

7. Serve the Spiced Lentil and Pumpkin Stew hot, garnished with fresh cilantro if desired.

Cabbage and Sausage Stew:

Ingredients:

- 1 lb smoked sausage, sliced
- 1 small head of cabbage, chopped
- 1 onion, finely chopped
- 3 cloves garlic, minced
- 2 carrots, peeled and sliced
- 2 potatoes, peeled and diced
- 1 can (14 oz) diced tomatoes
- 6 cups chicken or vegetable broth
- 1 teaspoon dried thyme
- 1 teaspoon caraway seeds (optional)
- Salt and pepper to taste
- 2 tablespoons olive oil
- Fresh parsley for garnish (optional)

Instructions:

1. In a large pot, heat olive oil over medium heat. Add sliced sausage and cook until browned.

2. Add chopped onion and garlic to the pot. Sauté until the onions are translucent.

3. Stir in chopped cabbage, carrots, and potatoes. Cook for a few minutes until the vegetables begin to soften.

4. Pour in the chicken or vegetable broth and diced tomatoes (with their juice). Add dried thyme and caraway seeds if using. Season with salt and pepper to taste.

5. Bring the stew to a simmer, then reduce the heat to low, cover, and let it simmer for about 20-25 minutes or until the vegetables are tender.

6. Taste and adjust the seasoning if necessary.

7. Serve the Cabbage and Sausage Stew hot, garnished with fresh parsley if desired.

Salmon and Potato Stew:

Ingredients:

- 1 lb salmon fillets, skin removed and cut into bite-sized pieces
- 4 potatoes, peeled and diced
- 1 onion, finely chopped
- 2 carrots, peeled and sliced
- 2 celery stalks, diced
- 3 cloves garlic, minced
- 1 can (14 oz) diced tomatoes
- 4 cups fish or vegetable broth
- 1/2 cup dry white wine (optional)
- 1 teaspoon dried dill
- 1 teaspoon paprika
- Salt and pepper to taste
- 2 tablespoons olive oil
- Fresh parsley for garnish (optional)
- Lemon wedges for serving

Instructions:

1. In a large pot, heat olive oil over medium heat. Add chopped onion, garlic, carrots, and celery. Sauté until the vegetables are softened.

2. Add diced potatoes to the pot and cook for a few minutes until they start to soften.

3. Pour in the fish or vegetable broth, diced tomatoes (with their juice), and white wine if using. Stir to combine.

4. Season the stew with dried dill, paprika, salt, and pepper. Mix well.

5. Bring the stew to a simmer, then reduce the heat to low, cover, and let it simmer for about 15-20 minutes or until the potatoes are tender.

6. Gently add the salmon pieces to the pot, ensuring they are submerged in the liquid. Simmer for an additional 5-7 minutes or until the salmon is cooked through.

7. Taste and adjust the seasoning if necessary.

8. Serve the Salmon and Potato Stew hot, garnished with fresh parsley if desired, and accompanied by lemon wedges for a burst of citrus flavor.

Quinoa and Vegetable Ratatouille:

Ingredients:

- 1 cup quinoa, rinsed
- 1 eggplant, diced
- 1 zucchini, diced
- 1 yellow squash, diced
- 1 bell pepper (any color), diced
- 1 onion, finely chopped
- 3 cloves garlic, minced
- 1 can (14 oz) diced tomatoes
- 2 tablespoons tomato paste
- 2 teaspoons dried thyme
- 2 teaspoons dried oregano
- Salt and pepper to taste
- 3 tablespoons olive oil
- Fresh basil for garnish (optional)

Instructions:

1. Cook quinoa according to package instructions. Set aside.

2. In a large skillet or pot, heat olive oil over medium heat. Add chopped onion and garlic. Sauté until the onions are translucent.

3. Add diced eggplant, zucchini, yellow squash, and bell pepper to the skillet. Cook for about 10 minutes, stirring occasionally, until the vegetables start to soften.

4. Stir in diced tomatoes (with their juice) and tomato paste. Mix well.

5. Season the vegetables with dried thyme, dried oregano, salt, and pepper. Stir to combine.

6. Cover the skillet or pot, reduce the heat to low, and let the Ratatouille simmer for about 15-20 minutes, or until the vegetables are tender.

7. Taste and adjust the seasoning if necessary.

8. Serve the Quinoa and Vegetable Ratatouille over a bed of cooked quinoa, garnished with fresh basil if desired.

Barley and Mushroom Stew:

Ingredients:

- 1 cup pearl barley, rinsed
- 2 cups mushrooms (button or cremini), sliced
- 1 onion, finely chopped
- 3 cloves garlic, minced
- 2 carrots, peeled and diced
- 2 celery stalks, diced
- 1 parsnip, peeled and diced
- 1 can (14 oz) diced tomatoes
- 6 cups vegetable broth
- 2 tablespoons tomato paste
- 1 teaspoon dried thyme
- 1 teaspoon dried rosemary
- Salt and pepper to taste

- 3 tablespoons olive oil
- Fresh parsley for garnish (optional)

Instructions:

1. In a large pot, heat olive oil over medium heat. Add chopped onion and garlic. Sauté until the onions are translucent.
2. Add sliced mushrooms to the pot and cook until they release their moisture and start to brown.
3. Stir in diced carrots, celery, and parsnip. Cook for a few minutes until the vegetables begin to soften.
4. Pour in the vegetable broth, diced tomatoes (with their juice), and rinsed barley. Stir to combine.
5. Add tomato paste, dried thyme, dried rosemary, salt, and pepper to the pot. Mix well.
6. Bring the stew to a simmer, then reduce the heat to low, cover, and let it simmer for about 30-40 minutes or until the barley is tender.
7. Taste and adjust the seasoning if necessary.
8. Serve the Barley and Mushroom Stew hot, garnished with fresh parsley if desired.

Pork and Cabbage Stew:

Ingredients:

- 1.5 lbs pork shoulder or pork stew meat, cut into bite-sized pieces
- 1 small head of cabbage, shredded
- 1 onion, finely chopped
- 3 cloves garlic, minced
- 2 carrots, peeled and sliced
- 2 potatoes, peeled and diced
- 1 can (14 oz) diced tomatoes
- 4 cups beef or vegetable broth
- 1 teaspoon dried thyme

- 1 teaspoon smoked paprika
- Salt and pepper to taste
- 2 tablespoons olive oil
- Fresh parsley for garnish (optional)

Instructions:

1. In a large pot, heat olive oil over medium heat. Add chopped onion and garlic. Sauté until the onions are translucent.
2. Add pork pieces to the pot and cook until browned on all sides.
3. Stir in shredded cabbage, sliced carrots, and diced potatoes. Cook for a few minutes until the vegetables start to soften.
4. Pour in the beef or vegetable broth and diced tomatoes (with their juice). Stir to combine.
5. Season the stew with dried thyme, smoked paprika, salt, and pepper. Mix well.
6. Bring the stew to a simmer, then reduce the heat to low, cover, and let it simmer for about 30-40 minutes or until the pork is tender and the vegetables are cooked through.
7. Taste and adjust the seasoning if necessary.
8. Serve the Pork and Cabbage Stew hot, garnished with fresh parsley if desired.

CHAPTER 10: WEEKLY MEAL PLAN FOR MELANOMA SURVIVORS

Breakfast: Berry and Spinach Smoothie (Mixed berries, spinach, Greek yogurt, almond milk)

Ingredients:

- 1 cup mixed berries (strawberries, blueberries, raspberries)
- 1 cup fresh spinach leaves, washed
- 1/2 cup Greek yogurt
- 1 cup unsweetened almond milk
- 1 tablespoon honey or maple syrup (optional, for sweetness)
- Ice cubes (optional)

Instructions:

1. Add mixed berries, fresh spinach leaves, Greek yogurt, and almond milk to a blender.
2. If you desire a sweeter smoothie, add honey or maple syrup to the blender.
3. Blend all the ingredients until smooth and creamy. If the consistency is too thick, you can add more almond milk to reach your desired thickness.
4. Taste the smoothie and adjust sweetness if needed.
5. If you prefer a colder smoothie, you can add ice cubes to the blender and blend until the ice is crushed and the smoothie is chilled.
6. Pour the Berry and Spinach Smoothie into glasses and enjoy immediately!

Lunch: Quinoa and Chickpea Bowl with Tahini Dressing

Ingredients:

For the Bowl:

- 1 cup quinoa, rinsed

- 1 can (15 oz) chickpeas, drained and rinsed
- 1 cup cherry tomatoes, halved
- 1 cucumber, diced
- 1 red bell pepper, diced
- 1/4 cup red onion, finely chopped
- 1/4 cup fresh parsley, chopped
- 1 tablespoon olive oil
- Salt and pepper to taste

For the Tahini Dressing:

- 1/4 cup tahini
- 2 tablespoons lemon juice
- 2 tablespoons water
- 1 tablespoon olive oil
- 1 clove garlic, minced
- Salt and pepper to taste

Instructions:

1. Cook quinoa according to package instructions. Once cooked, fluff with a fork and let it cool.
2. In a large bowl, combine cooked quinoa, chickpeas, cherry tomatoes, cucumber, red bell pepper, red onion, and fresh parsley.
3. Drizzle olive oil over the bowl and toss the ingredients until well combined. Season with salt and pepper to taste.
4. In a small bowl, whisk together tahini, lemon juice, water, olive oil, minced garlic, salt, and pepper to create the dressing.
5. Drizzle the tahini dressing over the quinoa and chickpea mixture. Toss until the salad is evenly coated with the dressing.
6. Serve the Quinoa and Chickpea Bowl with Tahini Dressing in individual bowls or plates.

7. Optional: Garnish with additional fresh parsley or a sprinkle of sesame seeds for extra flavor and presentation.

Dinner: Baked Salmon with Lemon and Dill, Steamed Asparagus, Quinoa

Ingredients:

For the Baked Salmon:

- 4 salmon fillets (6 oz each), skin-on or skinless
- 2 tablespoons olive oil
- 2 tablespoons fresh lemon juice
- 1 tablespoon fresh dill, chopped
- Salt and pepper to taste
- Lemon slices for garnish

For the Steamed Asparagus:

- 1 bunch of asparagus, woody ends trimmed
- 1 tablespoon olive oil
- Salt and pepper to taste

For the Quinoa:

- 1 cup quinoa, rinsed
- 2 cups water or vegetable broth
- Salt to taste

Instructions:

1. Preheat the Oven: Preheat your oven to 400°F (200°C).
2. Prepare the Baked Salmon:
   - Place the salmon fillets on a baking sheet lined with parchment paper.
   - In a small bowl, mix olive oil, lemon juice, chopped dill, salt, and pepper.
   - Brush the salmon fillets with the lemon and dill mixture, ensuring they are well coated.
   - Place a slice of lemon on top of each fillet for added flavor.

- Bake in the preheated oven for 12-15 minutes or until the salmon is cooked through and flakes easily with a fork.

3. Prepare the Steamed Asparagus:
   - While the salmon is baking, steam the asparagus. Place asparagus spears in a steamer basket over boiling water.
   - Steam for 4-6 minutes or until the asparagus is tender but still crisp.
   - Drizzle with olive oil and season with salt and pepper.

4. Prepare the Quinoa:
   - In a saucepan, combine quinoa and water or vegetable broth. Bring to a boil.
   - Reduce heat, cover, and simmer for 15-20 minutes or until quinoa is cooked and water is absorbed.
   - Fluff quinoa with a fork and season with salt.

5. Assemble the Dish:
   - Divide the cooked quinoa among plates.
   - Place a portion of baked salmon on each plate.
   - Arrange steamed asparagus alongside the salmon.
   - Garnish with additional lemon slices and fresh dill.

6. Serve and Enjoy: Serve the Baked Salmon with Lemon and Dill, Steamed Asparagus, and Quinoa immediately. Enjoy this wholesome and flavorful meal!

Day 2:

Breakfast: Avocado and Berry Parfait (Greek yogurt, avocado, mixed berries)
Ingredients:
- 1 ripe avocado, peeled and mashed
- 1 cup Greek yogurt
- 1 cup mixed berries (strawberries, blueberries, raspberries)
- 2 tablespoons honey or maple syrup (optional, for sweetness)

- Granola for layering (optional)
- Mint leaves for garnish (optional)

Instructions:

1. Prepare the Avocado Layer:
   - In a bowl, mash the ripe avocado until smooth.
2. Prepare the Greek Yogurt Layer:
   - In another bowl, mix the Greek yogurt. If desired, you can add honey or maple syrup to sweeten the yogurt.
3. Assemble the Parfait:
   - In serving glasses or bowls, start with a layer of the mashed avocado at the bottom.
   - Add a layer of Greek yogurt on top of the avocado.
   - Place a layer of mixed berries on the yogurt.
   - Repeat the layers until the glasses are filled, finishing with a layer of berries on top.
4. Optional: Add Granola:
   - For added texture and crunch, you can sprinkle a layer of granola between the avocado, yogurt, and berry layers.
5. Garnish and Serve:
   - Optionally, garnish the top with mint leaves for a fresh touch.
6. Chill and Enjoy:
   - Refrigerate the parfait for at least 30 minutes to let the flavors meld and the parfait to chill.
7. Serve Cold:
   - Serve the Avocado and Berry Parfait cold.

Lunch: Lentil and Vegetable Soup, Whole Grain Crackers

Lentil and Vegetable Soup:

Ingredients:

- 1 cup dried green or brown lentils, rinsed
- 1 onion, finely chopped
- 2 carrots, peeled and diced
- 2 celery stalks, diced
- 3 cloves garlic, minced
- 1 zucchini, diced
- 1 can (14 oz) diced tomatoes
- 6 cups vegetable broth
- 1 teaspoon ground cumin
- 1 teaspoon paprika
- 1 bay leaf
- Salt and pepper to taste
- 2 tablespoons olive oil
- Fresh parsley for garnish (optional)

Instructions:

1. In a large pot, heat olive oil over medium heat. Add chopped onion, carrots, celery, and garlic. Sauté until the onions are translucent.
2. Add diced zucchini to the pot and cook for a few minutes until it starts to soften.
3. Stir in rinsed lentils, diced tomatoes (with their juice), and vegetable broth. Mix well.
4. Season the soup with ground cumin, paprika, bay leaf, salt, and pepper. Stir to combine.
5. Bring the soup to a boil, then reduce the heat to low, cover, and let it simmer for about 25-30 minutes or until the lentils and vegetables are tender.
6. Taste and adjust the seasoning if necessary. Remove the bay leaf and discard.
7. Serve the Lentil and Vegetable Soup hot, garnished with fresh parsley if desired.

Whole Grain Crackers:

Ingredients:

- 1 cup whole wheat flour

- 1/4 cup olive oil
- 1/4 cup water
- 1/2 teaspoon salt
- 1/2 teaspoon dried herbs (such as rosemary or thyme), optional

Instructions:

1. Preheat the oven to 375°F (190°C).
2. In a bowl, combine whole wheat flour, olive oil, water, salt, and dried herbs if using.
3. Mix the ingredients until a dough forms. If the dough is too dry, you can add a little more water.
4. Roll out the dough on a floured surface to your desired thickness.
5. Cut the dough into cracker-sized pieces using a knife or a cookie cutter.
6. Place the crackers on a baking sheet lined with parchment paper.
7. Bake in the preheated oven for about 12-15 minutes or until the crackers are golden and crispy.
8. Allow the crackers to cool before serving.

Dinner: Turkey and Sweet Potato Skillet with Mixed Greens Salad

Turkey and Sweet Potato Skillet:

Ingredients:

- 1 lb ground turkey
- 2 sweet potatoes, peeled and diced
- 1 onion, finely chopped
- 2 cloves garlic, minced
- 1 teaspoon ground cumin
- 1 teaspoon smoked paprika
- 1/2 teaspoon ground cinnamon
- Salt and pepper to taste
- 2 tablespoons olive oil

- Fresh cilantro or parsley for garnish (optional)

Instructions:

1. In a large skillet, heat olive oil over medium heat. Add chopped onion and garlic. Sauté until the onions are translucent.
2. Add ground turkey to the skillet and cook until browned.
3. Stir in diced sweet potatoes, ground cumin, smoked paprika, ground cinnamon, salt, and pepper. Mix well.
4. Cover the skillet and let it simmer for about 15-20 minutes or until the sweet potatoes are tender, stirring occasionally.
5. Taste and adjust the seasoning if necessary.
6. Serve the Turkey and Sweet Potato Skillet hot, garnished with fresh cilantro or parsley if desired.

Mixed Greens Salad:

Ingredients:

- Mixed greens (such as spinach, arugula, and watercress)
- Cherry tomatoes, halved
- Cucumber, sliced
- Red bell pepper, sliced
- Balsamic vinaigrette dressing

Instructions:

1. In a large salad bowl, combine mixed greens, cherry tomatoes, cucumber, and red bell pepper.
2. Drizzle the salad with your favorite balsamic vinaigrette dressing. Toss gently to coat the greens.
3. Optional: Add a sprinkle of salt and pepper to taste.
4. Serve the Mixed Greens Salad alongside the Turkey and Sweet Potato Skillet.

Breakfast: Green Tea Chia Seed Pudding with Mango

Ingredients:

- 1/4 cup chia seeds
- 1 cup almond milk (or any milk of your choice)
- 1 green tea bag
- 1 tablespoon honey or maple syrup (optional, for sweetness)
- 1 ripe mango, peeled and diced
- Fresh mint leaves for garnish (optional)

Instructions:

1. Brew Green Tea:
   - Steep the green tea bag in hot water according to package instructions. Allow it to cool.
2. Make Chia Seed Pudding:
   - In a bowl, combine chia seeds and almond milk. Stir well to avoid clumps.
3. Add Green Tea:
   - Add the cooled brewed green tea to the chia seed mixture. Mix thoroughly.
4. Sweeten (Optional):
   - If you desire sweetness, add honey or maple syrup to the mixture and stir until well combined.
5. Refrigerate:
   - Cover the bowl and refrigerate the chia seed pudding for at least 3 hours or overnight. This allows the chia seeds to absorb the liquid and create a pudding-like consistency.
6. Assemble with Mango:
   - Once the chia pudding has set, layer it with diced mango in serving glasses or bowls.
7. Garnish:

o   Optionally, garnish the Green Tea Chia Seed Pudding with fresh mint leaves for a burst of flavor and presentation.

8. Serve:

    o   Serve the Green Tea Chia Seed Pudding with Mango chilled.

Lunch: Chickpea and Vegetable Mediterranean Salad

Ingredients:

- 1 can (15 oz) chickpeas, drained and rinsed
- 1 cucumber, diced
- 1 bell pepper (red, yellow, or orange), diced
- 1 cup cherry tomatoes, halved
- 1/2 red onion, finely chopped
- 1/2 cup Kalamata olives, pitted and sliced
- 1/2 cup crumbled feta cheese
- 1/4 cup fresh parsley, chopped

For the Dressing:

- 1/4 cup extra-virgin olive oil
- 2 tablespoons red wine vinegar
- 1 teaspoon dried oregano
- Salt and pepper to taste
- Optional: 1 clove garlic, minced

Instructions:

1. Prepare Chickpeas:

    o   If using canned chickpeas, drain and rinse them thoroughly.

2. Assemble Salad:

    o   In a large salad bowl, combine chickpeas, diced cucumber, diced bell pepper, cherry tomatoes, chopped red onion, Kalamata olives, crumbled feta cheese, and fresh parsley.

3. Make Dressing:

- In a small bowl, whisk together extra-virgin olive oil, red wine vinegar, dried oregano, salt, and pepper. If desired, add minced garlic for extra flavor.

4. Dress Salad:
   - Pour the dressing over the salad and toss gently until all ingredients are well coated.

5. Chill (Optional):
   - Refrigerate the salad for about 30 minutes to let the flavors meld and the salad to chill.

6. Serve:
   - Serve the Chickpea and Vegetable Mediterranean Salad as a refreshing side dish or a light main course.

Dinner: Mushroom and Spinach Stuffed Chicken Breast, Roasted Brussels Sprouts, Brown Rice

Ingredients:

- 4 boneless, skinless chicken breasts
- 1 cup mushrooms, finely chopped
- 2 cups fresh spinach, chopped
- 1/2 cup feta cheese, crumbled
- 2 cloves garlic, minced
- 1 teaspoon dried thyme
- Salt and pepper to taste
- Olive oil for cooking

Instructions:

1. Prepare the Filling:
   - In a pan, heat olive oil over medium heat. Add mushrooms and cook until they release their moisture.

- o Add minced garlic and chopped spinach to the pan. Cook until the spinach wilts.
    - o Stir in crumbled feta cheese, dried thyme, salt, and pepper. Cook for an additional 2 minutes, then remove from heat.
2. Prepare Chicken Breasts:
    - o Preheat the oven to 375°F (190°C).
    - o Butterfly each chicken breast by slicing horizontally through the middle, creating a pocket for the stuffing.
    - o Season the chicken breasts with salt and pepper.
3. Stuff Chicken Breasts:
    - o Stuff each chicken breast with the mushroom, spinach, and feta filling, pressing the edges to seal.
4. Cook Chicken:
    - o In an oven-safe skillet, heat olive oil over medium-high heat. Sear the stuffed chicken breasts on each side until golden brown.
    - o Transfer the skillet to the preheated oven and bake for about 20-25 minutes or until the chicken is cooked through.

Roasted Brussels Sprouts:

Ingredients:

- 1 lb Brussels sprouts, trimmed and halved
- 2 tablespoons olive oil
- Salt and pepper to taste

Instructions:

1. Preheat Oven:
    - o Preheat the oven to 400°F (200°C).
2. Prepare Brussels Sprouts:
    - o Toss halved Brussels sprouts with olive oil, salt, and pepper.
3. Roast Brussels Sprouts:
    - o Spread the Brussels sprouts on a baking sheet in a single layer.

o Roast in the preheated oven for about 20-25 minutes or until they are golden brown and crispy on the edges.

Brown Rice:

Ingredients:

- 1 cup brown rice
- 2 cups water or chicken broth
- Salt to taste

Instructions:

1. Cook Brown Rice:
   - In a saucepan, combine brown rice, water or chicken broth, and salt.
   - Bring to a boil, then reduce heat, cover, and simmer for 40-45 minutes or until the rice is cooked and water is absorbed.
2. Serve:
   - Serve the Mushroom and Spinach Stuffed Chicken Breast over a bed of brown rice with roasted Brussels sprouts on the side.
3. Enjoy:
   - Enjoy this wholesome and flavorful meal!

Day 4:

Breakfast: Spinach and Banana Protein Smoothie (Spinach, banana, protein powder, almond milk)

Ingredients:

- 1 cup fresh spinach leaves, washed
- 1 ripe banana
- 1 scoop vanilla protein powder
- 1 cup unsweetened almond milk
- Ice cubes (optional)

Instructions:

1. Prepare Ingredients:
   o Wash the fresh spinach leaves thoroughly.
   o Peel and slice the ripe banana.
2. Blend Ingredients:
   o In a blender, combine fresh spinach, sliced banana, vanilla protein powder, and unsweetened almond milk.
3. Optional: Add Ice Cubes:
   o If you prefer a colder smoothie, you can add ice cubes to the blender.
4. Blend Until Smooth:
   o Blend all the ingredients until smooth and creamy. If needed, you can adjust the consistency by adding more almond milk.
5. Taste and Adjust:
   o Taste the smoothie and adjust the sweetness or thickness by adding more banana or almond milk as desired.
6. Serve:
   o Pour the Spinach and Banana Protein Smoothie into a glass.

Lunch: Quinoa Minestrone Soup, Whole Wheat Roll

Quinoa Minestrone Soup:

Ingredients:

- 1 cup quinoa, rinsed
- 1 onion, finely chopped
- 2 carrots, peeled and diced
- 2 celery stalks, diced
- 3 cloves garlic, minced
- 1 zucchini, diced
- 1 can (14 oz) diced tomatoes
- 6 cups vegetable broth
- 1 can (15 oz) kidney beans, drained and rinsed

- 1 cup green beans, chopped
- 1 teaspoon dried oregano
- 1 teaspoon dried basil
- Salt and pepper to taste
- 2 tablespoons olive oil
- Fresh parsley for garnish (optional)
- Grated Parmesan cheese for serving (optional)

Instructions:

1. Prepare Quinoa:
   - Rinse quinoa under cold water. Set aside.
2. Sauté Vegetables:
   - In a large pot, heat olive oil over medium heat. Add chopped onion, carrots, celery, and garlic. Sauté until the onions are translucent.
3. Add Zucchini and Tomatoes:
   - Stir in diced zucchini and canned tomatoes (with their juice). Cook for a few minutes.
4. Pour in Broth:
   - Add vegetable broth to the pot. Bring the soup to a boil.
5. Add Quinoa and Beans:
   - Add rinsed quinoa, kidney beans, and chopped green beans to the pot. Stir well.
6. Season the Soup:
   - Season the soup with dried oregano, dried basil, salt, and pepper. Adjust seasoning to taste.
7. Simmer:
   - Reduce the heat to low, cover the pot, and let the soup simmer for about 15-20 minutes or until the quinoa is cooked and the vegetables are tender.
8. Garnish and Serve:

- o Garnish the Quinoa Minestrone Soup with fresh parsley and serve hot. Optionally, you can sprinkle grated Parmesan cheese on top.

Whole Wheat Rolls:

Ingredients:

- 2 cups whole wheat flour
- 1 tablespoon honey or maple syrup
- 1 packet (2 1/4 teaspoons) active dry yeast
- 3/4 cup warm water
- 1 tablespoon olive oil
- 1/2 teaspoon salt

Instructions:

1. Activate Yeast:
   - o In a small bowl, combine warm water, honey (or maple syrup), and yeast. Let it sit for 5-10 minutes until it becomes frothy.
2. Prepare Dough:
   - o In a large bowl, combine whole wheat flour, olive oil, and salt. Add the activated yeast mixture. Mix until a dough forms.
3. Knead and Rise:
   - o Knead the dough on a floured surface for about 5-7 minutes. Place the dough in a bowl, cover it, and let it rise in a warm place for 1-2 hours or until it doubles in size.
4. Shape Rolls:
   - o Preheat the oven to 375°F (190°C). Punch down the risen dough and shape it into small rolls.
5. Bake:
   - o Place the rolls on a baking sheet and bake in the preheated oven for 15-20 minutes or until they are golden brown.
6. Serve:
   - o Serve the Whole Wheat Rolls warm with the Quinoa Minestrone Soup.

Dinner: Grilled Chicken Caesar Salad with Whole Grain Croutons

Ingredients:

For the Grilled Chicken:

- 2 boneless, skinless chicken breasts
- 2 tablespoons olive oil
- 1 teaspoon garlic powder
- 1 teaspoon dried oregano
- Salt and pepper to taste
- Lemon wedges for serving

For the Caesar Salad:

- Romaine lettuce, washed and chopped
- 1/2 cup cherry tomatoes, halved
- 1/4 cup shaved Parmesan cheese
- Caesar dressing (store-bought or homemade)

For the Whole Grain Croutons:

- 2 cups whole grain bread, cut into cubes
- 2 tablespoons olive oil
- 1 teaspoon garlic powder
- 1 teaspoon dried thyme
- Salt and pepper to taste

Instructions:

1. Marinate and Grill Chicken:
   - In a bowl, mix olive oil, garlic powder, dried oregano, salt, and pepper. Coat the chicken breasts with the marinade and let them sit for at least 15 minutes.
   - Preheat the grill or grill pan over medium-high heat. Grill the chicken for about 6-8 minutes per side or until fully cooked. Slice the grilled chicken into strips.
2. Make Whole Grain Croutons:

o Preheat the oven to 375°F (190°C).

o Toss the bread cubes with olive oil, garlic powder, dried thyme, salt, and pepper. Spread them on a baking sheet.

o Bake in the preheated oven for about 10-15 minutes or until the croutons are golden and crispy.

3. Assemble Caesar Salad:

o In a large bowl, combine chopped romaine lettuce, halved cherry tomatoes, and shaved Parmesan cheese.

o Add the grilled chicken strips to the salad.

4. Add Croutons:

o Sprinkle the whole grain croutons over the salad.

5. Dress the Salad:

o Drizzle Caesar dressing over the salad. Toss the salad gently to coat all the ingredients evenly.

6. Serve:

o Divide the Grilled Chicken Caesar Salad among plates.

Day 5:

Breakfast: Turmeric Golden Milk Smoothie (Turmeric, banana, almond milk)

Ingredients:

- 1 ripe banana
- 1 teaspoon ground turmeric
- 1 cup unsweetened almond milk
- 1/2 teaspoon ground cinnamon (optional)
- 1/2 teaspoon honey or maple syrup (optional, for sweetness)
- Ice cubes (optional)

Instructions:

1. Prepare Ingredients:

o   Peel and slice the ripe banana.

2. Blend Smoothie:

    o   In a blender, combine the sliced banana, ground turmeric, almond milk, ground cinnamon (if using), and honey or maple syrup if you desire sweetness.

3. Optional: Add Ice Cubes:

    o   If you prefer a colder smoothie, you can add ice cubes to the blender.

4. Blend Until Smooth:

    o   Blend all the ingredients until smooth and well combined. Adjust the consistency by adding more almond milk if needed.

5. Taste and Adjust:

    o   Taste the smoothie and adjust sweetness or spice level according to your preference.

6. Serve:

    o   Pour the Turmeric Golden Milk Smoothie into a glass.

Lunch: Salmon and Kale Salad with Lemon Vinaigrette

Ingredients:

For the Salmon:

- 2 salmon fillets
- 1 tablespoon olive oil
- Salt and pepper to taste
- Lemon zest for garnish

For the Kale Salad:

- 4 cups kale, stems removed and leaves thinly sliced
- 1 cup cherry tomatoes, halved
- 1/2 cucumber, thinly sliced
- 1/4 cup red onion, thinly sliced
- 1/4 cup crumbled feta cheese (optional)

- 1/4 cup sliced almonds, toasted

For the Lemon Vinaigrette:

- 1/4 cup extra-virgin olive oil
- 2 tablespoons fresh lemon juice
- 1 teaspoon Dijon mustard
- 1 teaspoon honey or maple syrup
- Salt and pepper to taste

Instructions:

1. Prepare Salmon:
   - Preheat the oven to 400°F (200°C).
   - Place salmon fillets on a baking sheet. Drizzle with olive oil and season with salt and pepper.
   - Bake for 12-15 minutes or until the salmon is cooked through and flakes easily with a fork.
2. Make Lemon Vinaigrette:
   - In a small bowl, whisk together extra-virgin olive oil, fresh lemon juice, Dijon mustard, honey or maple syrup, salt, and pepper. Set aside.
3. Prepare Kale Salad:
   - In a large bowl, combine thinly sliced kale, cherry tomatoes, cucumber, red onion, and crumbled feta cheese (if using).
4. Toast Almonds:
   - In a dry pan over medium heat, toast sliced almonds until golden brown and fragrant. Be careful not to burn them.
5. Assemble Salad:
   - Drizzle half of the lemon vinaigrette over the kale salad and toss to coat the ingredients evenly.
6. Flake Salmon:
   - Once the salmon is done, flake it into bite-sized pieces.
7. Serve:

○ Divide the dressed kale salad among plates. Top with flaked salmon and toasted almonds.

Dinner: Quinoa and Vegetable Stir-Fry with Tofu

Ingredients:

For the Quinoa:

- 1 cup quinoa, rinsed
- 2 cups water or vegetable broth
- 1/2 teaspoon salt

For the Stir-Fry:

- 1 block firm tofu, pressed and cubed
- 2 tablespoons soy sauce or tamari
- 1 tablespoon sesame oil
- 1 tablespoon vegetable oil
- 3 cloves garlic, minced
- 1 tablespoon ginger, grated
- 1 red bell pepper, thinly sliced
- 1 carrot, julienned
- 1 zucchini, sliced
- 1 cup broccoli florets
- 1 cup snap peas, ends trimmed
- 2 green onions, sliced
- Sesame seeds for garnish (optional)

For the Sauce:

- 3 tablespoons soy sauce or tamari
- 2 tablespoons rice vinegar
- 1 tablespoon maple syrup or honey
- 1 teaspoon cornstarch mixed with 2 teaspoons water (for thickening)

Instructions:

1. Prepare Quinoa:
   - In a saucepan, combine quinoa, water or vegetable broth, and salt. Bring to a boil, then reduce heat, cover, and simmer for 15-20 minutes or until quinoa is cooked and water is absorbed. Fluff with a fork.
2. Marinate Tofu:
   - In a bowl, combine cubed tofu with soy sauce or tamari. Let it marinate for at least 15 minutes.
3. Cook Tofu:
   - In a large skillet or wok, heat vegetable oil over medium-high heat. Add marinated tofu cubes and cook until they are golden brown on all sides. Remove from the skillet and set aside.
4. Stir-Fry Vegetables:
   - In the same skillet, add sesame oil. Add minced garlic and grated ginger, sauté for about 30 seconds.
   - Add sliced bell pepper, julienned carrot, zucchini, broccoli florets, and snap peas. Stir-fry for 5-7 minutes or until the vegetables are crisp-tender.
5. Prepare Sauce:
   - In a small bowl, whisk together soy sauce or tamari, rice vinegar, maple syrup or honey, and the cornstarch-water mixture. Pour the sauce over the stir-fried vegetables.
6. Combine Tofu and Vegetables:
   - Add the cooked tofu back to the skillet with the vegetables. Toss everything together until well coated in the sauce.
7. Serve:
   - Serve the Quinoa and Vegetable Stir-Fry with Tofu over a bed of cooked quinoa.

Breakfast: Mixed Berry Overnight Oats (Rolled oats, mixed berries, almond milk)

Ingredients:

- 1/2 cup rolled oats
- 1/2 cup mixed berries (strawberries, blueberries, raspberries)
- 1/2 cup almond milk
- 1 tablespoon chia seeds (optional, for added thickness)
- 1 tablespoon maple syrup or honey (optional, for sweetness)
- Greek yogurt or additional berries for topping (optional)

Instructions:

1. Combine Ingredients:
   - In a jar or container, combine rolled oats, mixed berries, almond milk, chia seeds (if using), and maple syrup or honey (if desired).
2. Mix Well:
   - Stir the ingredients well to ensure the oats and berries are evenly distributed.
3. Refrigerate Overnight:
   - Cover the jar or container and refrigerate overnight or for at least 4 hours. This allows the oats to absorb the liquid and the flavors to meld.
4. Stir Before Serving:
   - Before serving, give the overnight oats a good stir to combine all the ingredients. If the mixture is too thick, you can add a little more almond milk to reach your desired consistency.
5. Optional Toppings:
   - Top the Mixed Berry Overnight Oats with a dollop of Greek yogurt or additional berries for extra freshness and flavor.
6. Serve and Enjoy:

o   Spoon the overnight oats into a bowl or eat directly from the jar. Enjoy this nutritious and convenient breakfast!

Lunch: Tuna and White Bean Salad, Whole Grain Crackers

Tuna and White Bean Salad:

Ingredients:

- 2 cans (5 oz each) canned tuna, drained
- 1 can (15 oz) white beans (cannellini or navy), drained and rinsed
- 1/2 red onion, finely chopped
- 1 cup cherry tomatoes, halved
- 1/4 cup Kalamata olives, pitted and sliced
- 1/4 cup fresh parsley, chopped
- 2 tablespoons capers, drained (optional)
- 2 tablespoons extra-virgin olive oil
- 1 tablespoon red wine vinegar
- Salt and pepper to taste
- Lemon wedges for serving

Instructions:

1. Prepare Tuna and Beans:
   - In a large bowl, combine drained tuna and white beans.
2. Add Vegetables:
   - Add finely chopped red onion, halved cherry tomatoes, sliced Kalamata olives, chopped fresh parsley, and capers (if using) to the bowl.
3. Make Dressing:
   - In a small bowl, whisk together extra-virgin olive oil and red wine vinegar. Season with salt and pepper to taste.
4. Combine and Toss:
   - Pour the dressing over the tuna and white bean mixture. Toss everything together until well combined.

5. Chill (Optional):

    ○ For enhanced flavors, cover the bowl and refrigerate the salad for about 30 minutes before serving.

6. Serve:

    ○ Serve the Tuna and White Bean Salad with lemon wedges on the side.

Whole Grain Crackers:

Ingredients:

- 1 cup whole grain flour
- 1/4 cup olive oil
- 1/4 cup water
- 1/2 teaspoon salt
- 1/2 teaspoon dried herbs (such as rosemary or thyme), optional

Instructions:

1. Preheat Oven:

    ○ Preheat the oven to 375°F (190°C).

2. Prepare Dough:

    ○ In a bowl, combine whole grain flour, olive oil, water, salt, and dried herbs if using. Mix until a dough forms.

3. Roll and Cut Crackers:

    ○ Roll out the dough on a floured surface to your desired thickness. Cut the dough into cracker-sized pieces using a knife or a cookie cutter.

4. Bake:

    ○ Place the crackers on a baking sheet lined with parchment paper.
    ○ Bake in the preheated oven for about 12-15 minutes or until the crackers are golden and crispy.

5. Cool and Serve:

    ○ Allow the crackers to cool before serving.

Dinner: Roasted Butternut Squash Soup, Grilled Chicken Breast

Roasted Butternut Squash Soup:

Ingredients:

- 1 medium-sized butternut squash, peeled, seeded, and diced
- 1 onion, chopped
- 2 carrots, peeled and chopped
- 2 cloves garlic, minced
- 2 tablespoons olive oil
- 4 cups vegetable or chicken broth
- 1 teaspoon ground cumin
- 1/2 teaspoon ground cinnamon
- Salt and pepper to taste
- 1/2 cup coconut milk (optional, for creaminess)
- Roasted pumpkin seeds for garnish (optional)
- Fresh parsley or cilantro for garnish (optional)

Instructions:

1. Roast Vegetables:
   - Preheat the oven to 400°F (200°C).
   - In a baking sheet, toss diced butternut squash, chopped onion, carrots, and minced garlic with olive oil. Roast for 25-30 minutes or until vegetables are tender and slightly caramelized.
2. Blend Soup:
   - Transfer the roasted vegetables to a blender. Add vegetable or chicken broth, ground cumin, ground cinnamon, salt, and pepper. Blend until smooth.
3. Heat and Add Coconut Milk (Optional):
   - Pour the blended soup into a pot. Heat over medium-low heat. If desired, stir in coconut milk for added creaminess. Adjust seasoning to taste.
4. Serve:

o Ladle the Roasted Butternut Squash Soup into bowls.

5. Garnish:

   o Garnish with roasted pumpkin seeds and fresh parsley or cilantro if desired.

Grilled Chicken Breast:

Ingredients:

- 2 boneless, skinless chicken breasts
- 1 tablespoon olive oil
- 1 teaspoon paprika
- 1/2 teaspoon garlic powder
- Salt and pepper to taste
- Lemon wedges for serving

Instructions:

1. Marinate Chicken:

   o In a bowl, mix olive oil, paprika, garlic powder, salt, and pepper. Coat the chicken breasts with the marinade and let them marinate for at least 15 minutes.

2. Grill Chicken:

   o Preheat a grill or grill pan over medium-high heat. Grill the chicken breasts for about 6-8 minutes per side or until fully cooked.

3. Rest and Slice:

   o Let the grilled chicken rest for a few minutes before slicing it into thin strips.

4. Serve:

   o Serve the Grilled Chicken Breast alongside the Roasted Butternut Squash Soup.

5. Squeeze Lemon:

   o Squeeze fresh lemon juice over the grilled chicken for added brightness.

Breakfast: Almond Butter and Banana Whole Wheat Toast

Ingredients:

- 2 slices whole wheat bread
- 2 tablespoons almond butter
- 1 ripe banana, sliced
- Honey for drizzling (optional)
- Chia seeds or sliced almonds for garnish (optional)

Instructions:

1. Toast the Bread:
   - Toast the slices of whole wheat bread to your desired level of crispiness.
2. Spread Almond Butter:
   - While the bread is still warm, spread a generous layer of almond butter evenly on each slice.
3. Add Banana Slices:
   - Arrange the sliced banana on top of the almond butter, covering the entire surface of the toast.
4. Drizzle Honey (Optional):
   - If you desire extra sweetness, drizzle a bit of honey over the banana slices.
5. Garnish (Optional):
   - Optionally, sprinkle chia seeds or sliced almonds on top for added texture and nutritional benefits.
6. Serve:
   - Place the Almond Butter and Banana Whole Wheat Toast on a plate and serve immediately.

Lunch: Avocado and Shrimp Salad with Citrus Vinaigrette

Ingredients:

For the Salad:

- 1 lb large shrimp, peeled and deveined
- 2 avocados, diced
- 1 cup cherry tomatoes, halved
- 1 cucumber, diced
- 1/4 red onion, thinly sliced
- Mixed salad greens (lettuce, arugula, or spinach)

For the Citrus Vinaigrette:

- 1/4 cup extra-virgin olive oil
- 2 tablespoons fresh orange juice
- 1 tablespoon fresh lemon juice
- 1 teaspoon Dijon mustard
- 1 teaspoon honey or maple syrup
- Salt and pepper to taste

Optional Garnish:

- Fresh cilantro or parsley, chopped
- Sesame seeds or poppy seeds

Instructions:

1. Cook Shrimp:
   - In a pan, cook the shrimp over medium heat until they are pink and opaque, about 2-3 minutes per side. Set aside.
2. Prepare Salad Ingredients:
   - In a large salad bowl, combine diced avocados, halved cherry tomatoes, diced cucumber, thinly sliced red onion, and mixed salad greens.
3. Make Citrus Vinaigrette:
   - In a small bowl, whisk together extra-virgin olive oil, fresh orange juice, fresh lemon juice, Dijon mustard, honey or maple syrup, salt, and pepper.

4. Assemble Salad:
   - Add the cooked shrimp to the salad ingredients in the bowl.
5. Drizzle with Citrus Vinaigrette:
   - Drizzle the citrus vinaigrette over the salad and shrimp. Toss gently to coat everything in the dressing.
6. Garnish (Optional):
   - Optionally, garnish the salad with fresh chopped cilantro or parsley and sprinkle sesame seeds or poppy seeds on top.
7. Serve:
   - Serve the Avocado and Shrimp Salad immediately.

Dinner: Vegetable and Lentil Curry with Brown Rice

Ingredients:

For the Vegetable and Lentil Curry:

- 1 cup dry brown lentils, rinsed and drained
- 1 large onion, finely chopped
- 2 cloves garlic, minced
- 1 tablespoon ginger, grated
- 1 can (14 oz) diced tomatoes
- 1 can (14 oz) coconut milk
- 3 cups mixed vegetables (such as carrots, bell peppers, zucchini, and peas)
- 2 tablespoons curry powder
- 1 teaspoon ground turmeric
- 1 teaspoon ground cumin
- 1 teaspoon ground coriander
- 1/2 teaspoon chili powder (adjust to taste for spice level)
- Salt and pepper to taste
- 2 tablespoons cooking oil
- Fresh cilantro for garnish

For the Brown Rice:

- 1 cup brown rice
- 2 cups water
- Pinch of salt

Instructions:

1. Cook Brown Lentils:
   - In a medium-sized pot, combine rinsed brown lentils with water. Bring to a boil, then reduce heat, cover, and simmer for about 20-25 minutes or until lentils are tender but still hold their shape. Drain any excess water.
2. Prepare Brown Rice:
   - In a separate pot, combine brown rice, water, and a pinch of salt. Bring to a boil, then reduce heat, cover, and simmer for about 40-45 minutes or until rice is cooked and water is absorbed.
3. Sauté Onion, Garlic, and Ginger:
   - In a large skillet or pot, heat cooking oil over medium heat. Add finely chopped onion and sauté until translucent. Add minced garlic and grated ginger, sauté for an additional minute.
4. Add Spices:
   - Stir in curry powder, ground turmeric, ground cumin, ground coriander, and chili powder. Cook for 1-2 minutes until fragrant.
5. Add Vegetables:
   - Add diced tomatoes, coconut milk, mixed vegetables, and cooked brown lentils to the pot. Stir well to combine.
6. Simmer:
   - Bring the mixture to a simmer, then reduce heat and let it simmer for about 15-20 minutes until the vegetables are tender and the flavors meld.
7. Season:
   - Season the curry with salt and pepper to taste. Adjust the spice level if needed.

8. Garnish and Serve:
    - Garnish the Vegetable and Lentil Curry with fresh cilantro. Serve over cooked brown rice.

Afternoon Snack: Carrot Sticks with Hummus

Ingredients:

- 4-5 medium-sized carrots, peeled and cut into sticks
- 1 cup hummus (store-bought or homemade)
- Fresh parsley or cilantro for garnish (optional)
- Olive oil for drizzling (optional)
- Paprika for sprinkling (optional)

Instructions:

1. Prepare Carrot Sticks:
    - Wash, peel, and cut the carrots into sticks, ensuring they are of uniform size for even dipping.
2. Make or Prepare Hummus:
    - You can either make your own hummus or use store-bought hummus. If making your own, blend chickpeas, tahini, garlic, lemon juice, olive oil, and salt until smooth.
3. Arrange Carrot Sticks:
    - Arrange the carrot sticks on a serving platter or plate.
4. Serve with Hummus:
    - Place the hummus in a bowl or a small serving dish alongside the carrot sticks.
5. Garnish (Optional):
    - Optionally, garnish the hummus with a drizzle of olive oil, a sprinkle of paprika, or fresh chopped parsley or cilantro.

6. Serve and Enjoy:
    - ○ Serve the Carrot Sticks with Hummus as a healthy and tasty snack or appetizer.

Evening Snack: Greek Yogurt with Honey and Almonds

Ingredients:

- 1 cup Greek yogurt
- 2 tablespoons honey (adjust to taste)
- 2 tablespoons almonds, sliced or chopped
- Fresh mint leaves for garnish (optional)

Instructions:

1. Prepare Greek Yogurt:
    - ○ Scoop 1 cup of Greek yogurt into a serving bowl.
2. Drizzle with Honey:
    - ○ Drizzle 2 tablespoons of honey over the Greek yogurt. Adjust the amount of honey to your desired level of sweetness.
3. Add Almonds:
    - ○ Sprinkle sliced or chopped almonds over the yogurt and honey.
4. Garnish (Optional):
    - ○ Optionally, garnish with fresh mint leaves for a burst of freshness.
5. Serve and Enjoy:
    - ○ Serve the Greek Yogurt with Honey and Almonds immediately and enjoy this simple, protein-packed, and satisfying snack or breakfast.

Beverages:

Throughout the Day: Infused Water (Cucumber and Mint)

Ingredients:

- 1 medium cucumber, thinly sliced

- Handful of fresh mint leaves
- 1-2 liters of water (depending on your container size)
- Ice cubes (optional)

Instructions:

1. Prepare Ingredients:
   - Wash the cucumber thoroughly and slice it into thin rounds.
   - Wash the mint leaves and pat them dry.
2. Assemble Infusion Jar or Pitcher:
   - In a large jar or pitcher, combine the cucumber slices and fresh mint leaves.
3. Add Water:
   - Pour 1-2 liters of water over the cucumber and mint in the jar or pitcher. Adjust the quantity based on your preference and the size of your container.
4. Infuse:
   - Let the water infuse with the flavors of cucumber and mint. For a stronger flavor, refrigerate the infused water for at least 2 hours, or preferably overnight.
5. Serve:
   - When ready to serve, you can strain the water to remove the cucumber and mint pieces, or you can leave them in for visual appeal.

Between Meals: Green Tea or Herbal Infusions

Ingredients:

- 1 tea bag of green tea or herbal tea of your choice (e.g., chamomile, peppermint, hibiscus)
- 1 cup water (8 ounces, boiling)

Optional Additions:

- Honey or agave syrup for sweetness
- Lemon slices or a splash of lemon juice
- Fresh herbs (mint, basil) for added flavor

- Slices of ginger or a cinnamon stick for warmth

Instructions:

1. Boil Water:
   - Boil 1 cup of water. Allow it to cool slightly for a moment after boiling.
2. Prepare Tea Bag:
   - Place the tea bag of your choice into a teapot or a heat-resistant mug.
3. Pour Water Over Tea Bag:
   - Pour the hot water over the tea bag, ensuring it is fully submerged.
4. Steep the Tea:
   - Let the tea bag steep in the hot water. The recommended steeping time varies based on the type of tea:
     - Green tea: 2-3 minutes
     - Herbal tea: 5-7 minutes (or as per package instructions)
5. Optional Additions:
   - If desired, add honey or agave syrup for sweetness, lemon slices or juice for a citrusy touch, fresh herbs for added flavor, or slices of ginger or a cinnamon stick for warmth.
6. Remove Tea Bag:
   - Once the tea has steeped to your liking, remove the tea bag from the water.
7. Strain (Optional):
   - If you've added loose herbs or spices, you may want to strain the tea as you pour it into your cup.
8. Serve: Pour the infused tea in a mug or cup.

CREATING A MELANOMA-FRIENDLY KITCHEN

1. Invest in Colorful Fruits and Vegetables:

   Fill your refrigerator with a rainbow of colorful fruits and vegetables high in antioxidants. Berries, leafy greens, carrots and tomatoes are examples of foods that may benefit overall skin health.

2. Select Lean Proteins:

Choose lean proteins like fish, poultry, tofu, and lentils. These give important nutrients without including significant amounts of saturated fat.

3. Include Omega-3-Rich Foods:

Keep omega-3-rich items in your cabinet such as fatty fish (salmon, mackerel) flaxseeds, chia seeds and walnuts. Omega-3 fatty acids may be anti-inflammatory.

4. Staple Whole Grains:

To add fiber and critical nutrients to your meals, use whole grains such as brown rice, quinoa and whole wheat pasta.

5. Herbs and spices can be used:

Incorporate a variety of herbs and spices to boost flavor without relying on excessive salt. Anti-inflammatory qualities are found in turmeric, ginger and garlic for example.

6. Cooking Oils that are Good for You:

Keep healthy cooking oils on hand such as olive oil which includes monounsaturated fats and antioxidants. Consider avocado oil or coconut oil for many cooking purposes.

7. Incorporate Nuts and Seeds:

Keep a variety of nuts and seeds on hand for snacking or incorporating into dishes. Healthy fats and nutrients can be found in almonds, walnuts, chia seeds and sunflower seeds.

8. Limit your intake of processed foods:

Reduce the availability of processed foods and snacks high in added sugars and harmful fats. Choose whole, less processed foods.

9. Dairy Alternatives or Low-Fat Dairy:

To limit saturated fat intake choose low-fat or substitute dairy products. Consider almond milk or Greek yogurt as alternatives.

10. Station of Hydration:

Make sure you have a continual supply of water in your kitchen. It is critical to stay hydrated for overall health and skin hydration.

11. Organize for Convenience:

Arrange your kitchen such that healthful products are easily accessible. In the pantry and refrigerator, keep fruits, veggies and whole grains at eye level.

12. Containers for Meal Prep:

Invest in meal prep containers to make portioning and storing healthy meals easier. This can save time while also encouraging portion management.

13. Reading Labels is a Habit:

Make it a practice to read food labels. Look for items with as little additives, preservatives and hidden sugars as possible.

14. Snacks for the Sun:

Include snacks high in vitamins C and E which may help with skin health. For a sun-safe snack, consider citrus fruits, almonds and seeds.

15. Environment for Mindful Eating:

Set aside time for meals, limit distractions and savor the flavors of your melanoma-friendly dishes to create a mindful eating environment.

CHOOSING HEALTHY COOKING METHODS

1. Grilling:

Grilling is a healthy cooking method that imparts a smoky flavor to foods without excessive added fats. Opt for lean proteins like fish, chicken, or vegetables.

2. Baking:

Baking is a versatile and low-fat cooking method. It preserves the natural flavors of ingredients without the need for excessive oils or fats.

3. Steaming:

Steaming is a gentle cooking method that retains the nutrients in foods. Steam vegetables, fish, or poultry to maintain their natural goodness.

4. Roasting:

Roasting brings out rich flavors by caramelizing the natural sugars in foods. Use this method for vegetables, lean meats, or whole grains.

5. Sauteing:

Sautéing involves cooking food quickly in a small amount of oil. Choose heart-healthy oils like olive or avocado oil and pair with colorful vegetables or lean proteins.

6. Poaching:

poaching involves cooking food in simmering liquid, preserving its natural flavors. Try poaching fish or eggs for a light and healthy meal.

7. Slow Cooking:

Slow cooking allows ingredients to simmer and develop deep flavors without excessive added fats. It's an excellent method for stews, soups, and lean meats.

8. Pressure Cooking:

Pressure cooking retains nutrients due to shorter cooking times. Use a pressure cooker for beans, whole grains, or stews.

9. Griddling:

Griddling, or cooking on a flat surface, requires minimal oil. Use a griddle for cooking vegetables, lean meats, or whole-grain pancakes.

10. Broiling:

Broiling is a cooking method that exposes food to direct heat. It's great for quickly cooking lean proteins like chicken or fish.

11. Microwaving:

Microwaving is a quick and efficient way to cook or reheat food. It requires little to no added fats, making it a healthy option for certain dishes.

12. Stir-Frying:

Stir-frying involves cooking small, bite-sized pieces of food quickly in a small amount of oil. Opt for colorful vegetables and lean proteins.

13. Blanching:

Blanching briefly cooks food in boiling water and then immediately places it in ice water to stop the cooking process. It's ideal for vegetables, preserving their color and nutrients.

14. Smoking:

Smoking is a flavorful cooking method that imparts a unique taste to foods. It's often used for lean proteins like fish or poultry.

15. Using Herbs and Spices:

Enhance the flavor of your dishes without relying on excessive salt or unhealthy fats by incorporating a variety of herbs and spices. They add depth and richness to your meals.

EXERCISE AND ITS ROLE IN MELANOMA CARE

1. Immune System Aid:

Exercise on a regular basis has been linked to a stronger immune system. A strong immune system is essential for defending the body and may aid in melanoma prevention and treatment.

2. Improved Circulation:

Exercise improves blood circulation, ensuring that oxygen and nutrients are distributed properly to all cells, including skin cells. Improved circulation benefits skin health in general.

3. Reducing Stress:

Exercise is a natural stress reliever assisting in the management of stress levels which can have an impact on general well-being. Lowering stress levels may help to improve immunological function.

4. Weight Control:

Maintaining a healthy weight is critical in melanoma treatment. Regular exercise paired with a healthy diet can aid in weight management and lower the risk of obesity-related problems.

5. Synthesis of Vitamin D:

Outdoor activities expose the body to sunlight, which aids in vitamin D synthesis. Adequate vitamin D levels have been linked to a lower risk of developing various malignancies including melanoma.

6. Increased Sleep Quality:

Regular physical activity helps to improve sleep quality. Sleep is critical for overall health and may improve the body's ability to repair and rejuvenate.

7. Function of the Lymphatic System:

Exercise promotes the proper operation of the lymphatic system which aids in immunological function. This can help the body locate and eradicate cancerous cells.

8. Better Mood and Mental Health:

Regular exercise releases endorphins, which improves mood and mental well-being. Positive mental health is critical in dealing with a melanoma diagnosis.

9. Muscle Function and Strength:

Muscle strength must be maintained through training for total physical function. This is especially critical for people undergoing melanoma treatments which can impair strength and movement.

10. Cancer Rehabilitative Care:

Exercise can be used into cancer rehabilitation programmes to assist patients in regaining strength, endurance and overall function following melanoma therapies.

11. Inflammation is reduced:

Chronic inflammation has been linked to an increased risk of a variety of diseases including cancer. Exercise contains anti-inflammatory properties that may benefit general health.

12. Social Assistance:

Participation in group workouts or activities allows for social connection and support. Emotional well-being is an important element of melanoma treatment.

13. Physical Activities in the Sun:

To reduce sun exposure engage in sun-safe physical activities. Outdoor activities should be done in the early morning or late afternoon and protective clothes and sunscreen should be worn.

www.ingramcontent.com/pod-product-compliance
Lightning Source LLC
Chambersburg PA
CBHW050805260726
48660CB00004B/1261